M000189659

SHIFTING GEARS

SHIFTING GEARS

From Anxiety and Addiction to a Triathlon World Championship

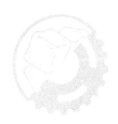

ADAM HILL

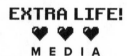

EXTRA LIFE!
♥ ♥ ♥
M E D I A

SHIFTING GEARS
From Anxiety and Addiction to a Triathlon World Championship

ISBN   978-1-5445-2585-3   *Hardcover*
       978-1-5445-2583-9   *Paperback*
       978-1-5445-2584-6   *Ebook*

CONTENTS

Fear and Loathing in a Mexican Porta Potty

IRONMAN LOS CABOS, 2014. MILE 133.

This was not how I expected things to turn out.

I was doubled over in a porta potty in downtown San Jose del Cabo. I felt a combination of intense pain, lightheadedness, exhaustion, and gastric chaos. As I reflected back on what brought me to this uncomfortable moment, I realized I only had myself to blame. I signed up for this, and despite my current shameful circumstances, I was about to achieve absolute glory. Well, as much glory as one can achieve in soiled Lycra. Before I could achieve said glory, though, I had to survive the present situation.

The lightheadedness worried me most. The last thing I wanted was for some tourist to pop open the blue plastic door and discover a gringo passed out with his shorts around his ankles and covered in his own sick.

Keep it together, man! Head between your knees. Breathe in, breathe out...

The afternoon heat of Cabo intensified within the big blue hot box, producing an unbearable fecal humidity. I knew full well that my bare ass was in contact with the most unsanitary of toilet seats. In any other circumstance, I would have relied on my quadriceps to hold me in a squatting position to avoid any contact with the seat in question, or I would have lined the seat with some toilet paper. But neither was an option in this instance. The need for immediate rest and relief took priority over personal hygiene. Time was of the essence. This was not my finest moment.

Toilet paper...Oh, fuck! I hope there's toilet paper in here!

I glanced over, panicked. Toilet paper was on the roll. Thank God. I could go back to my pity party and the thoughts running through my head.

What the hell am I doing here?

I want to quit so bad.

I can't quit; I'm almost there.

"Almost there" is eight more miles! Fuck this!

Don't pass out.

Shape up, man! When you finish this thing, it's going to be glorious! There will be pizza!

Pizza? Are you serious? I feel like shit right now!

Despite my miserable state, things could have been a lot worse. The porta potty was my refuge. Ten minutes before, when my stomach dropped and it was clear that I would not be able to trust my bowels to cooperate from that point forward, I had a desperate need for release. It was the culmination of a week's worth of anxiety, more than five hundred grams of sugar consumed on the racecourse, and probably some bad Mexican tap water. For two miles, I tried to hold it in, but with each new step, I found myself on the verge of failure. At the instant I was ready to squat behind a cactus, I came upon an oasis in the desert: this porta potty. It was a shining, smelly beacon in the darkness of panic and urgency.

When I fell through the spring-loaded door to my place of refuge, I felt instant relief. This was followed immediately by the realization that I was about to succumb to heatstroke. The temperature outside was about 85 degrees, but this dirty sauna had to be 120 degrees. All of the liquid in my body became sweat in an instant; my heart rate surged, and my blood pressure dropped.

All of this led me to sitting in the porta potty with my head between my knees, struggling to stay conscious, and asking myself why on earth I would ever subject myself to this type of torture.

The irony of finding myself in this situation was not lost on me. Here I was at mile eighteen of a marathon after a 2.4-mile swim and a 112-mile bike ride in the Mexican desert. I was as sick as a dog and in a pretty shameful state. I was racing in an Ironman to prove how *healthy and fit* I was, but this experience was oddly reminiscent of my days as a heavy drinker—hugging toilet seats, passing out in random places, and suffering from what alcoholics call "incomprehensible demoralization."

I thought of all the times my alcohol abuse hurt my family. I thought of the shame and humiliation it brought them. I thought of myself dying at an early age, unable to see my daughter and son graduate from high school and college. I thought of how I used to wake up full of fear and anxiety, forced to fake it through the day until I could finally drink my liquid solution.

Thinking through where I had been brought my perspective back to a positive place. I had been sober for two years in that moment. A little over a year before this race, I quit smoking, put down the junk food, and got my unhealthy ass off the couch. Despite having no athletic prowess whatsoever, I became inspired to compete in Ironman Triathlons. Having achieved a dramatic spiritual and psychological transformation through sobriety, I wanted to make a similar physical transformation. But my ultimate goal was not just to finish an Ironman—I wanted to compete at the top of the world stage. I wanted to qualify for the Ironman World Championship. This was my first attempt at achieving that goal, and while it wasn't going quite to plan, the journey to the starting line led to the transformation I wanted to achieve and became a catalyst for transcending my fears.

During this moment, sitting on a porta potty in San Jose del Cabo at mile 133 of my first Ironman Triathlon, I didn't feel like much of a champion. I was closer to the edge of giving up. Thankfully, I remembered why I began in the first place. Outside that blue plastic door was a little less than eight more miles of a race I began a year prior. At the end of those final eight miles was the greatest finish line in the world, and proof positive that I accomplished what I had set out to do.

I pulled myself up, yanked up my triathlon shorts, took another deep breath of the microscopic fecal humidity, and exited my place of refuge. Once again, I was off and running.

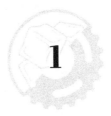

BUDGIE
SMUGGLERS

was thirteen years old the first time I wore a Speedo. Thirteen is the exact age that a boy should *not* wear a Speedo. No human being wants to see a puberty-stricken man-boy at the height of awkwardness wearing what can only be described as 90 percent polyester, 10 percent nylon, and 100 percent "nope." Whoever does should probably be arrested.

Yet there I was, one week before my first day of high school, sitting in my mom's Dodge Caravan with nothing but a towel covering my shame. I stared anxiously at the entrance to the high school pool, trying to muster enough courage to go in. My head swiveled, looking for other kids with the same level of fear in their eyes. The only thing that would give me any semblance of comfort was the knowledge that somebody was feeling the same level of shame and embarrassment that I was.

All I needed was one poor fool to appear more insecure than I was. That would reinforce that I was not alone. I could easily blend in and not draw any attention to myself while the other poor sucker bore all the humiliation.

My mom finally broke the silence and asked the obvious question, "Well? Are you going to go try out for this water polo team or not?"

Why am *I here?* I thought to myself. Somehow the idea seemed grand when it was first presented to me. But now? Not so much. As the tight elastic began to ride up my butt crack, I started second-guessing my initial enthusiasm.

Two weeks earlier, during high school registration, a nice administrator asked me if there were any activities I wanted to try in the fall semester. Water polo did not immediately come to mind. In fact, nothing came to mind. I believe it was the impromptu staring contest and the ensuing awkwardness that prompted the registration lady to suggest I try water polo. Because I was a scrawny, slow-to-develop spaz-fest with zero friends who was consumed with the fear of ridicule and physical pain, you might be wondering why I would want to join a sport where I was required to don nut-huggers and nearly drown at the hands of the jockiest of all jocks in Jockland. Many years later, I still wonder the same thing. Yet, I nodded. Water polo it was.

"Well?" my mom asked after not getting an immediate response.

I thought for a second before I answered. I glanced down at the towel, which covered my chicken legs. I felt the constraint of the banana hammock around my nether regions as I pondered my high school destiny. On one hand, I could grit my teeth and overcome this pulsating anxiety, open the car door, and walk to the pool, where I would remove my towel and expose my thirteen-year-old, bright-white body in nothing but a German marble bag. This would be my first exposure to high school life.

On the other hand, I could feel the sweet and immediate relief of quitting before I even started. I could tell my mom I wasn't interested in water polo anymore. I could just join regular PE instead. Nobody ever got picked on in PE...ever.

I, of course, chose the latter. I embraced the immediate euphoria of pain and humiliation avoidance. I enabled my fearful nature, and for one more day, I was safe. My weenie bikini was stored in the bottom of my underwear drawer for the rest of my teens, and my mom was mildly irritated that she had to drive all the way to the high school at six in the morning for nothing.

Taking the easy way out and avoiding risks was nothing new to me. Throughout much of my childhood, I steadily learned that behavior. I would aspire to do something great, face ridicule from my peers, and then decide to give up. Fear was a constant driver in any decision I made, and it slowly and silently imprinted itself into my psyche early in life.

I grew up in Southern California in a small town called Dana Point. The town itself was relatively sleepy and was once famous as a killer surf spot. Killer Dana, as the lineup was called, was rendered extinct in the late sixties by the construction of a boat harbor. The surfers who objected to the construction of the harbor were entirely ignored, and the local stuffed shirts literally dropped boulders on their once pristine surf spot. The community became something new entirely, a dichotomy of wealthy executives and retirees blended with "just scraping by" sailors, surfers, and working-class families. For most of my youth, my family fell into the latter category.

My great-grandfather, C. B. Hill, was the first in the Hill family to put down roots in Southern California. He started a small business in Los Angeles in 1923, and it's still a family business in its fourth generation. My father was an employee of the Northern California branch when I was born. Two years later, he was transferred to an operations position down south where he would split his working hours between East Los Angeles and Anaheim, California. Desiring a safe home for his family and proximity to the ocean, he moved us into a small, three-bedroom house in Dana Point, enduring the daily one- to two-hour commute each way.

I was fortunate to have a father who cared deeply enough to move us to Dana Point and a mother who chose to stay at home and take care of my siblings and me. I recognized how lucky I was to have two parents who still loved each other and cared for their family, especially during a time when divorce was becoming a theme in many families.

Both of my parents had been married previously. From those marriages, my dad had a son and my mom had a son and a daughter. My parents met one another at the family business, where my mom was a receptionist. After they married, I came along a little over a year later, and our family was complete.

I enjoyed being the youngest of four siblings by more than six years. For the most part, because I was so much younger, the older kids kept to themselves, and I felt more like an only child in a home full of adults. Even though I was a young child during the eighties, my house was full of teenagers, so I felt like I experienced the eighties as a teenager. I was constantly barraged with music from The Cure or Talking Heads, movies like *The Breakfast Club*, and every other piece of eighties pop culture. They were formative for my psyche and later blissfully nostalgic.

Because I had the influence of older siblings, I found it difficult to relate to my elementary school peers. I was terribly afraid of confrontation. I also lacked any prowess in the arena of ball sports. This was a tragic combination for a young boy that made me develop into something of a spaz. Some of the other kids quickly discovered my spazzy essence, and like sharks tasting a drop of spaz-laden blood, they exploited my weakness. I knew I couldn't gain their respect through brute force, so I became a class clown as a way to earn favor. One desperate tactic I employed to try to impress the other kids was to purposely mispronounce words during reading time to make them sound vulgar or humorous. If I was asked to read a passage that said, "The settlers removed the goods from the chuck wagon," I'd instead read aloud "chick wagon," to the absolute delight of my peers. This obviously came at the expense of my grades and likely (despite my intentions) at the expense of any respect from the other children. While they were laughing, it's clear to me now that they weren't laughing with me.

The social relationships I had in elementary school had their ups and downs. At times, I felt welcomed by some of the kids, but more often than not, I felt like a bit of an outcast, clinging on to social relationships out of desperation more than any real connection. Most of the friends I had tolerated me at best, and I was often subjected to the typical verbal bullying of the time. I had my share of run-ins with bullies.

Instances where I actually stood up for myself were few and far between, but I did have a few brief moments of courage. Once, a kid started tripping me from behind while we were standing in line. He found my clumsiness hilarious. The physical torment was annoying to be sure, but it was the humiliating (and unfortunately completely accurate) insults that drove me over the edge. He called me out on one of my most embarrassing traits—bedwetting.

Being a bedwetter until roughly the age of ten never served my social status very well. I rarely went to sleepovers, but when I did, it was impossible to hide my shame. There's only so many times I could "accidentally" spill water that happened to smell like urine all over my sleeping bag. Unsurprisingly, the few so-called friends who did find out about this exploited this information freely with my fellow classmates. Such was the case on that day.

Finally, after I was tripped from behind one too many times, I turned around and passively pushed the kid back. Taking this as a challenge, he asked, not so politely, if I would care to engage in fisticuffs. I think his exact words were, "Do you want your ass kicked?" Hoping to avoid immediate punishment from the teacher standing ten feet away from us, we agreed to meet on the playground after school, as if we were in an early-eighties, coming-of-age, after-school special on the importance of standing up to a bully.

Now, it's important to note that I had never been in a fight before. I had been on the receiving end of sucker punches, pantsings, and plenty of embarrassing physical assaults, but never a fistfight. I suspect the reason I had never been in a fight was *not* because all of the kids feared me and my lightning-fast Bruce Lee karate fists. On the contrary, I never got into a fight because I spent my entire life trying to *avoid* fighting. I had become an expert at swallowing my pride and taking "option X" when the choice was "do X, or I'll kick your ass!"

I knew my place. Plus, I had a low tolerance for physical pain. But that day was different. I was done being pushed around. I was done with fair-weather friends, being made fun of for my awkwardness, and putting up with physical and verbal abuse. I made a decision to stand up for myself and face my bully.

Until I got home.

I remember arriving at home from school before the fight was to take place and my mom saying that she was going to the store and that she didn't want me to go anywhere. That's when the strangest thing happened. Either by divine intervention or my own subconscious fear trying to protect me from harm,

I forgot that I had a fight scheduled. I guess I forgot to put it on my calendar.

How something so big and looming could simply be lost in a fit of absentmindedness, I will never know, but I only discovered my mistake when I received a knock on the door that afternoon. When I answered the door, one of my classmates was standing there.

"Um...Are you going to come fight that one kid?" he asked sheepishly.

"Oh yeah! I guess I forgot about that," I replied. "Well, I can't now because my mom's not home, and she asked me not to go out."

I may as well have handed him nails and a hammer and stepped inside my own coffin.

He looked at me and smirked as if he had just gained some powerful piece of information that would make the entire school praise him as a divine prophet when he imparted this knowledge upon them. He skipped away, armed with his new-found popularity, and I didn't give it a second thought. I simply went back to watching the *Animaniacs*.

The next day, I was met with ridicule the likes of which I had never experienced before. Kids shoved me as I walked toward my desk, calling me all sorts of unrepeatable names. As we stood for the Pledge of Allegiance, my desk mate punched me so hard in the stomach that I doubled over and had to sit down. The teacher immediately yelled at me for sitting during the pledge, causing the eyes of every student to fall upon me as I held my stomach and cried.

My embarrassment was so great that I asked for a hall pass to see the school nurse. As I left the class, one final insult was hurled, "That's right! Run away again, pussy!"

It's what I always did. I ran away.

It was a painful and humiliating experience at the time, but looking back, I get a small sense of satisfaction that I wasted the afternoon of twenty or so blood-thirsty adolescents and basically conveyed to my adversary that he really just wasn't worth my time.

As I approached junior high, the few kids who I had surrounded myself with had become bored with me, and I found myself alone most school days. While I had some acquaintances, I never took any initiative to make new friends. I opted instead to keep to myself and avoid all the conflict and rejection that I knew would come from immersing myself in the social world of junior high. If I could keep my nose clean and head down, perhaps I would make it through these torturous two years. It was the safe option, but it also cemented in me a social anxiety that persisted well into adulthood. Keeping to myself, while maintaining relative safety, didn't really cultivate any self-esteem. I didn't think very much of myself and began to develop a sense of worthlessness. I experienced very little emotional development during those years. In fact, I likely regressed.

Throughout this period of my life, because of the aforementioned spazziness and fear of risk-taking, I participated in activities at a mediocre level, opting to remain solely in my comfort zone. I had enjoyed surfing since about the age of seven, but I rarely ventured away from the gentle waves of Doheny Beach to explore more advanced breaks. I was afraid that the powerful surf would end my life, or worse, I would be given grief by the locals. I played baseball, but I never progressed because I was afraid of being hit by a pitch or dropping a ball and letting everyone down.

I even tried my hand at football. The idea of wearing pads and a helmet excited my adolescent male brain. My imagination conjured up fantasies of me evading the tackles of prepubescent gladiators to score game-winning touchdowns. I even had my hopes stirred up by former professional football player Roger Staubach.

One weekend, word made it around our neighborhood that Roger Staubach was filming a promotional video at our local high school football field. I decided to visit the field in hopes of getting a glimpse of the former superstar quarterback.

Since I had just joined the Mission Viejo Cowboys football team, I put on my jersey and shorts, along with a pair of knee-high crew socks, grabbed my football, and headed to the high school. I wanted to give the impression that I was only there to run some football drills, not bother the poor man who was trying to work.

I arrived at the field and wandered over toward the crowd of onlookers. During a break in filming, I caught Mr. Staubach's attention. He gave me a curious squint when he noticed the football under my arm. He looked at me, and his hands popped up into the universal signal for, "Hey! Throw me the ball!"

I nearly shit myself, but I obliged and promptly tossed the ball straight over his head, completely missing the clear and sizeable target he was making between his hands. He leaped and awkwardly fell backward as he tried to catch the wayward ball. He recovered, picked the ball up, and threw a perfect spiral back to me. I proceeded to play catch with Mr. Staubach between takes for the next hour.

The experience had a lasting impression on me. Even at my young age, I was able to grasp the amazing example this man was setting as a public figure. He didn't have to play catch with me, but he understood that he could make a significant impact by doing so.

After the impromptu game of catch, he signed my ball "To Adam: Star of the future," and posed for a picture with me. Since the picture was taken with Mr. Staubach's own camera, I didn't think that I would ever see it. A few days later at lunch, a school administrator came up to my table holding a glossy photograph.

"A man came into our office and asked me to deliver this to you," she said. It was the picture of Roger Staubach and me. He found out where I went to school and hand delivered the photo.

I was blown away. What a class act. The experience fired me up. I was now convinced that football was my destiny and that I would be a star just as Mr. Staubach had said. At practice over the course of the following weeks, reality proved to be much different. Despite the kind and encouraging words of a professional football player, it was clear I did not have the hand-eye coordination to play ball sports. Furthermore, the gridiron is not a place for a kid who is afraid of being hit. Fear quickly began to overshadow my enthusiasm for the sport.

One particular drill terrified me the most. All of the players gathered in a large circle with the coach in the middle. The athletes banged their helmets, beat their chests, and hoot and hollered while the coach scanned the group for victims. He chose two players to face one another a few feet apart within the circle. As the rhythmic hubbub intensified, the coach shouted, "Go!" At that point the two athletes lunged toward each other at full speed, meeting in the middle with a huge crash. There was no clear winner in this exercise, and the only purpose I presume that it served was to get the players used to getting hit very hard.

For me, it only served to increase my aversion to being hit. I dreaded being chosen to enter the circle. One occasion cemented my decision to quit football forever and never look back. The coach rested his gaze upon me and told me to step forward. My stomach immediately dropped, and I was overcome with terror. The terror only intensified when the coach chose my opponent: the biggest, meanest player on the team.

The other player burst into the circle, intensity in his eyes, teeth gritting rabidly. I did nothing to hide how intimidated I was, which only fueled his fury. I fought back tears as the energy of the crowd intensified, and then heard the coach yell, "Go!" All I could do was shut my eyes and brace for the collision. I immediately felt the impact of my opponent's helmet against my belly, quickly followed by the impact of my back to the ground. For a few moments, I struggled to breathe through the intense pain in my gut. The coach approached me and gave me a quick and pitiful look.

"Looks like you got the wind knocked outta ya, Hill," he said. "Why don't you sit out the rest of the practice?"

I did as the coach ordered, and took it a step further, never returning to another practice.

The general themes of my young life were avoidance, quitting, and fear of failure. I was so full of fear that I chose to live a life of mediocrity and isolation instead of taking risks and potentially get hurt or laughed at.

But what if I *did* do something great? What if I actually tried something and found out that it was exhilarating and life-affirming? The idea never crossed my mind. I was so resigned to fear that the concept of actually being a hero never entered my mind. My brain predetermined that I was a guaranteed failure, so I might as well avoid the pain of trying. Any potential pleasure associated with a successful risk was not reward enough for me to overcome the overwhelming fear of failure, rejection, and hurt.

Junior high became a two-year period of slipping into and out of shadows to avoid attention. I was constantly afraid I might be noticed and held up as a loser to be ridiculed and torn down. I was anxious whenever I was in a social situation, and in my mind, I was not good at anything. If there was any silver lining to this self-isolation, it was that I mostly escaped bullies. I knew I was a prime target, so I stayed away from almost anyone. And it worked.

Following the years of isolation in middle school, I entered high school desperate for connection, despite my preconditioned fears. I was vulnerable and highly impressionable. I felt lonely and starved for acceptance and kinship—a necessary element for survival as a human being. At the point in life when a person's identity starts to take shape, I felt like I had no identity.

That longing for acceptance brought me to the parking lot of the high school in my Speedo. But the fear I developed over my entire childhood kept me from opening the car door and taking the next step. My habits were too strong at that point to overpower.

During the first few weeks of high school, I was a piece of clay to be molded by any group who would take me in. Really, it could have been anybody with any intentions. Fortunately, the person who let me in would become one of my greatest influences and would ultimately save my life.

Bryn sat with the "safe" crowd. When I say "safe," I mean they didn't pose any danger of punching me in the face or inflicting any significant social humiliation. These were kids who were generally too interested in academics and roleplaying games to waste any time tormenting their peers.

Translation: these were the nerds.

Even though I didn't necessarily live up to the academic qualifications of the group, I was able to earn my seat through an awkward and childish sense of humor. This was the catalyst by which Bryn and I became fast friends. He and I shared the same sense of humor. More than that, we shared a brain. We were like platonic soulmates and generally spent most of our free time together.

Bryn was different in a few ways, but this didn't cause conflict. They were complementary differences, especially from my perspective. I aspired to have the traits that Bryn had and I lacked.

For example, Bryn had far more confidence than me in most respects. In fact, he was brimming with confidence in every area. If he had a test to take, there was no need to study; he would just go in and ace the damn thing. He wanted to learn how to play guitar, so he went and did it. He became one of the best guitarists I've known. It wasn't because of some freakish natural ability; it was because when he told himself that he could do something, he believed it to his core, and it became true with the right amount of work. This, I would come to learn later, is a common characteristic among most, if not all, high-performing individuals. I envied his confidence from the first day I met him.

It even extended to relations with girls I liked, which was something else I lacked entirely. Many of my conversations with girls started (and ended) like this:

Me to incredibly intimidating girl: "Hey. What's...'sup?"

Incredibly intimidating girl: "Hi, Adam! Not much. What's up with you?"

Me: "Good."

As sad as this sounds, I deserved the embarrassment. The truth is that when a girl did express an interest in me, I suddenly became disinterested, mostly because of fear. I had a fear of intimacy and vulnerability. When things got serious, I jumped ship. Thus, my awkward relationship with girls. I would become quietly obsessed with a girl (such was my nature) while at the same time becoming aloof at any speck of interest expressed in me. All the while, I would have a pity party that I couldn't get a girlfriend.

What. A. Dick.

Some of Bryn's confidence did rub off on me, however. Music became my outlet. I played cello from the age of nine, but I never really dedicated much effort to it. I usually sat in the last row, last chair, shadow-bowing my way to invisible stardom. Then I realized that I would need a plan to get into college.

While my grades were acceptable, they were by no means impressive to any college. Sports weren't going to get me there. I tried out for the basketball team (since there was minimal concern with getting hurt, and no Speedos), but I was one of only two players cut during tryouts. That's right. The coaches only cut two players, and I was one of them. The team that I didn't make went on to a stellar 2–8 season.

I made the baseball team by some miracle, but I sat on the bench most of the year and watched our junior varsity team lose every single game they played. Not that I would have helped. I rarely, if ever, hit the ball outside of the infield.

I opted to skip baseball to participate in the exciting world of high school drumline—a PE credit I was able to earn despite never actually banging a stick against a drum in a competition.

This was a benefit of earning some leverage with my newfound cello skills. My music teacher mercifully looked the other way at my lack of attendance and gave me an A nonetheless.

Music became my gateway to greater self-confidence and purpose. It also became my therapy. Once I chose to apply myself, I practiced two to three hours per day and excelled very quickly. Cello was one of the few areas of my life where I had any confidence. I enjoyed the feeling that I was the best at something. It gave me a sense of purpose during a time when I was aimlessly wandering around. I realized that I craved a feeling of excellence and thrived on personal development.

My vast and rapid improvement with the cello was my first indication that I could learn and apply things very quickly if I chose to focus on them. I didn't know it at the time, but it was the first manifestation of an obsessive personality, a trait that would be a source of tremendous trouble for me, but would also become a superpower. When my freshman year ended, I was the last chair cellist. When I came back in the fall, I auditioned my way to first chair. I started auditioning for various orchestras around California. I made it into the All-Southern California High School Orchestra and then into the All-State High School Orchestra.

My tremendously good fortune in finding a friend like Bryn was the catalyst to turning my social life around. I went from a complete social outcast to a marginally accepted awkward teenager. Look out, George Jefferson, because I was movin' on up!

Bryn and I made names for ourselves on the high school newspaper, where we were self-proclaimed editors of the humor page. Our brand of humor was a balance of highbrow and obscene. The highbrow stuff was mostly in the form of inside jokes hidden in top ten lists (a tradition started by our predecessors and David Letterman) and puns that went over the heads of our fellow students. The obscene stuff rarely made it past the filter of our no-nonsense journalism teacher. Still, it made me proud to be a part of something that was not only fun and enriching but also made me feel accepted.

With music being such an influential part of my young life, as well as Bryn's, we did what every teenager with a bent toward music and a narrow view of the world chooses to do. We set out to become famous rock stars. At about the same time Bryn began teaching himself the guitar, I did the same, and we began to write some songs. Enlisting the skills of Bryn's brother on bass and a mutual friend on drums, we had our first band, The Clap.

The entire purpose of our first band name was so that if we were ever booked for a gig (we weren't), we could post flyers that read "Catch The Clap this Saturday at The Tavern!"

Less grotesquely, this name was also a nod to one of my first influences in rock and roll, Eric Clapton. I tried to model much of my musical stylings around Clapton and other blues musicians of the time. Of course, the resulting songs showed every bit of my sixteen years. The first song I ever wrote was a twelve-bar blues song called "Yo Mama's a Ho," which I would belt out in the vocal style of B. B. King.

The Clap didn't last long, maybe a few months. Our sensibilities evolved and we devised a new, more sophisticated band name: The Mojo Wire. The blues and surf influence remained, but we introduced an indie rock component to our songwriting. We didn't go very far, even in our local music scene, but it was fun, and at the time, that was all that mattered.

Having these friends made me feel secure, comfortable, and confident. Yet there was a lingering social anxiety. On days where I found myself alone or not able to play music, I felt depressed. I still felt as though I was facing the constant judgment of my classmates, and their opinions of me mattered way too much in my mind.

Overall, my high school life was extremely positive. My grades flourished, I evolved as a musician, I was coming out of my shell (aside from my terrible fear of girls), and I had a great core group of friends. As we approached the time to begin applying to colleges, I continued to sharpen my musical resume to ensure my success in getting into a school of my choice. In my final year of high school, I auditioned for and performed with the Pacific Symphony Institute, a program for gifted musicians. I also entered into, and won, a variety of music competitions.

I would have never considered auditioning for honors orchestras or entering music competitions if not for my private teacher, Joan Lunde. Somehow, she saw something in me that I didn't see within myself, and she enabled me to express myself through music and flourish in that world. There is no doubt that I was fortunate to have her guidance in my life.

Many teachers or coaches simply followed a curriculum instead of training the individual. Joan seemed to recognize that practicing endless technique without context would neither motivate nor drive me. She saw that I had passion and emotion to convey, and music could be a vessel to deliver it. Of course, I still had to work on technical skills, but they were presented in such a way that I knew how they would contribute to my goal: to project my passion through art.

I knew Joan had a desire to challenge me when, early in our time together, she placed a piece of music in front of me. There were a lot of notes on this piece of music...a lot. The name of the composer was foreign to me also. My knowledge of classical music was shallow at best, so I knew of Mozart, Beethoven, and Tchaikovsky, but the name Camille Saint-Saëns was obscure to me.

But I was about to become very familiar with Mr. Saint-Saëns. I was about to learn his cello concerto, and if I could do so successfully, it would become my ticket to college.

Joan then pulled out a vinyl album from her shelf and put it on the record player. Following the obligatory scratch, I heard a powerful single quarter note played by a string orchestra, followed by a powerful single quarter note played by a solo cellist. Following that quarter note (the easiest note in the piece) came a series of fast triplets melded together, melodies played high on the neck of the instrument, and very technical staccato sections.

In a word, the piece was intimidating.

"You want me to play this?" I asked her. I assumed she had this piece reserved for one of her star cellists.

"This piece suits you," she said simply, her words accompanied by a confident smirk.

She then took the piece of music and began marking it up with a pencil as if she were grading a dissertation.

"I want you to practice each of these sections ten times, slowly and with perfect form," she instructed.

I did as she said, practicing very slowly and deliberately using the best technique I could. The results were remarkable. Within a few sessions of consistent and slow work, I mastered the sections, one by one. Chunking the sections down into bite-sized parts and practicing them very slowly over and over again made the task much less intimidating and far more achievable.

I would later discover that training slow with great technique and consistency would become a recipe for success in my life.

Within a matter of weeks, I had mastered the piece to a level that I could play it at recitals, competitions, and auditions. Eventually, it helped me earn a scholarship to the University of California, Santa Barbara (UCSB).

A number of very accomplished professional cellists credit Ms. Lunde with being a significant influence on their development. Her unique approach to my style of learning led to my success with the instrument.

Getting into UCSB was a dream come true. The campus sat right on the Pacific Ocean, which was an important draw for me. I couldn't imagine a more beautiful place to spend the next few years of my life.

The last few months of high school were blissful. I had discovered a passion for music, and I had good friends, despite the lingering social anxiety. I was eager to start my next chapter in my new beautiful home of Santa Barbara, a place that could only be described as heaven.

Little did I know I would spend the next few years believing I was in hell, a place where I could look around and see so much peace and beauty yet experience so much despair. It was in Santa Barbara that internal torment would redevelop and consume me. It was where I would lose control of my life and become everything I hated. It was there that I would discover what seemed to be a solution to my social phobias, fears, and anxieties—but instead was a "solution" that would become its own problem. It was a problem that would nearly ruin my life and the lives of those I loved.

The Cannon

IRONMAN LOS CABOS, 2014.
T-MINUS TEN MINUTES TO START. MILE 0.

Oh, man. I'm already starting to sweat. This is not good.

I put on my wetsuit too early, wanting to get a practice swim in before the start of the race. Now, I was standing on the shoreline in the start corral and sweating beneath a layer of thick neoprene designed to keep my body warm in cold water. The water temperature today was seventy-five degrees, and as the sun peeked over the horizon, the coolness of the morning was quickly transforming into an oppressive heat.

I hadn't even started the race yet, and the fear of dehydration was already at the front of my mind. No drinkable water was nearby. The next available water station would only come after 2.4 miles of swimming.

Can I last for over an hour before getting any fresh drinking water in me? What if I overheat and pass out during the swim? What if the seawater causes me to dehydrate more quickly?

These were all baseless fears anxiety created in my head as I walked toward the start line of my first Ironman, in Los Cabos, 2014. There was nothing to fear. This feeling was just the remnants of the obsessive, fearful person I once was, the person who lost control over fear. I wasn't the person who feared being uncomfortable, who would quit rather than endure any uncomfortable experiences. Compromising my goals or sense of accomplishment for the safer option was all behind me. I just needed to find enough proof to convince my brain I was right and anxiety was wrong. So I looked around. Seeing the hundreds of other racers standing in their wet-suits before me made me realize that all was right with the world. I was about to become an Ironman, come what may.

A sea of calm flooded over me. I knew I had this.

Boom!

The calm turned to chaos as eight hundred athletes rushed toward the turquoise waters of Palmilla Beach. Far to the right and in the middle of the pack, I found myself rushing with them until we met the water with a crash and our arms took over for our legs.

We flailed along like fish caught in a net, each trying to find our own small piece of ocean that we could call our own. Each athlete, as if fighting for survival, thrashed toward that first turn buoy.

As we made a left turn, four hundred yards into the swim, the space opened up as we began the long, two-kilometer stretch parallel to the shore. The seafloor began to disappear into a dark blue abyss. I had found my place, my rhythm, and my home for the next hour. Solitude.

2

The Dysfunctional
Love Affair

lcohol was my solution for all the anxiety-inducing
negative thoughts and baseless fears constantly flooding my brain. I knew it the first time that I tried it. At
seventeen years old, I sat in a cliffside shack on Del Playa Road
in the college town of Isla Vista with a red cup in my hand that
was one-fourth Mickey's Lager and three-fourths foam. My body
responded with a gag upon my first sip, but my brain shouted a
resounding "YES!" to the feeling. Two and a half more red cups
later, I had a wonderful buzz and was the life of the party. At
about midnight, I walked back to my friend's dorm room with
zero consequences, and I fell asleep with a smile on my face.

It was the perfect first experience with alcohol. The very
first sip was a revelation. I now had a solution to fear. My social
anxieties, my awkwardness around others, my anger, and my
worry all dissolved like the foam atop the red Solo cup. It was

all washed away with the warm elixir flowing through my veins and numbing my pain.

That was the experience that sold me on UCSB. It wasn't the only reason I chose this school, but the promise of reliving that experience again sealed the deal for me. After that first visit to UCSB, and until I moved there permanently, I seldom drank alcohol again. It wasn't something I craved or felt I needed. I wasn't white-knuckling my way through high school until I could once again get my hands on booze. It was simply a social elixir, and an effective one at that.

Since I never felt any cravings, only the subtle realization that alcohol removed my social phobias, I had no reason to suspect that I would one day be a problem drinker. In fact, I didn't even know what that was. In my naïveté, I assumed alcoholism and addiction were things reserved for degenerates and deplorables. It was a conscious choice made by bad people or people with traumatic backgrounds, not people who had ambition, intelligence, and morality. I had never even known an alcoholic, nor had I seen that many people drink to intoxication. Growing up, I was surrounded by "normies." The party at UCSB was really my first experience at a party where people were drinking in excess, and every single one of them looked happier because of it. There were no bad people here that I could see. Just people having a good time.

Had I known at the time that I would be a problem drinker, maybe I wouldn't have tried it...or maybe I would have tried it anyway, thinking that I would somehow be able to manage it. That's the odd thing about alcoholism. An alcoholic doesn't really know they're an alcoholic until they're in the grips of alcoholism...and then it's too late.

After graduating high school, I proceeded to have the best three months a teenager could have. The summer of 1997 was the summer of zero consequences. The summer before I left for college imprinted in me the grand idea of what drinking should be—euphoric, carefree, and everlasting. I never blacked out, never got sick, never got a hangover, and never got out of hand—well, never got *seriously* out of hand. I could drink with friends and wake up early the next morning to go to work, productive as ever. I did this while watching my friends suffer through massive hangovers. I felt like I was built for drinking.

I was in the safety of friends' homes, their parents away on business or vacation, leaving their oversized Orange County homes unoccupied for their quasi-responsible teenage children to oversee. It was the perfect opportunity for fifteen to twenty eighteen-year-olds to run rampant in togas throughout the backyard as they pounded shitty beer, which had no other purpose than to be chugged as quickly as possible.

At one party in particular, two friends and I entered into a drinking contest. The prize? Nothing but pride. Within an hour, I was ping-ponging between two bathrooms, taking care of those two friends as they traded off between passing out and violently vomiting into and around the toilet. Later in the evening, I attended to another friend who was vomiting all over himself in the backyard. The only words I could understand from him were, "Hose me down!" Of course, I promptly obliged.

It's important to note that I wasn't *sober* at these times. I was in fact drinking just as much as the others. The difference was that, for some strange reason, these first experiences with drinking just made me feel good and confident, not sick or out of control.

We had these parties almost weekly. Feeling buzzed and surrounded by friends was a stark contrast to the introversion and loneliness I felt throughout most of my adolescence. It wasn't hard for me to associate alcohol with the joy I was experiencing. In reality, however, it wasn't the alcohol; it was being surrounded by people I loved that gave me meaningful joy. Alcohol just magnified the feeling of acceptance and belonging. I was subconsciously creating the perverted belief that alcohol was causing it. Throughout my drinking career, these were the experiences I obsessively chased in vain.

When I left for college, the party continued. If I were asked what I was good at during my early college days, I would have answered "drinking." While athleticism and academics didn't necessarily come naturally to me, drinking did. It was something I looked forward to and began to focus on while I lost focus on things that were once beautiful to me, like music.

As I ventured into the new world of college, the feeling of joy, ambition, and purpose I had experienced over the previous few years quickly faded into the past. I began to feel lost as I stepped out of my comfort zone of South Orange County into a new place with new faces, new experiences, and no direction. The cello, which had been my salvation in high school, began to take a backseat. I had achieved my goal of getting into college, and I didn't see much of a future with it, so I lost the drive that consumed me in high school. I had little direction, and it began to manifest as a steadily growing internal depression. I found myself pining for the past, wanting to get away from this new place with new experiences that were outside of my comfort zone and go back to the place where I was safe. At home.

It was a strange and subtle depression that I didn't understand. I knew that I was lucky to be in my situation. I knew I lived in the most amazing place where opportunities were around every corner, and I was deeply frustrated that I couldn't enjoy that. I tried to force myself to appreciate the world I was occupying. I tried surfing, walking in nature, and taking day trips with friends, but none of it popped that bubble of sadness. I saw my friends enjoying themselves, finding direction, and excelling in their courses, but I was struggling and falling into mild—and gradually deeper—despair.

I found some solace in a nightly cigarette with friends outside of my dorm. One cigarette turned into two, which turned into five, and finally became half a pack a day. It was immediate relief from my depression, but it took an obvious toll on my health. I was sick more often, tired all the time, and didn't want to leave my bed.

After one experience where I became lightheaded and fainted while filling up a soda in the dining commons, I went to the doctor. He diagnosed me with mononucleosis, the "kissing disease," without much investigation. There was no lab work; we just had a five-minute interview, an assessment of my vitals, and a half-assed diagnosis. I think my condition was probably just sadness mixed with increasingly unhealthy habits.

Then there was alcohol. Just the action of popping a bottle cap off induced a Pavlovian response of relief from the depression. It was like a switch had suddenly flipped in my brain, and I was back to normal. The life of the party.

It was under this cloud of depression that I officially ended my cello career at UCSB, a choice that should have taken much more time and consideration. In my state, however, the choice seemed obvious. Unfortunately, the curse of hindsight and experience reveals the enormity of my mistake. I gave up something that provided joy and fulfillment. It was the vessel that held all of my hopes and dreams and a positive outlet for my obsessive nature. After walking away from it, I no longer had that outlet.

There was only drinking.

Drinking heavily in the town of Isla Vista was not uncommon, so excessive drinking did not stand out the way it might have in other places. An alcohol problem, in an environment rife with abundant alcohol consumption and debauchery, can be easily mistaken for normal behavior. If there was a problem, it would go unnoticed until it was too late. Even as my control began to wane, my ability to "handle" alcohol was lauded by my peers, and I saw it as a talent. It was an enabling environment, to say the least.

My ignorance to my budding drinking problem was reinforced by a few factors. For one, everyone else in my sphere was doing it. Additionally, I never craved it. It simply existed as the weekend activity of choice. If a weekend went by where I didn't drink, my world wasn't destroyed. The only subtle clue that it could be a problem was that it numbed my pain, removed my worry, and brought me out of the fog of depression. While I recognized that it was a solution to my problems, the realization was so subtle and my knowledge so limited that I never would have connected the dots to create a picture of a problem drinker. The elation and joy, along with the minimal consequences, fostered an obsession that I didn't anticipate—an insidious descent into alcoholism.

The challenge, of course, was obtaining the alcohol. This was a problem mitigated simply by knowing the right people, having access to those people, and being within proximity to an establishment that would sell large quantities of alcohol to these people without judgment. Fortunately for us, we lived in Isla Vista, a place where these factors worked together in harmony. I was rarely in want of my solution.

The arrangement came together perfectly my sophomore year of college when I met "the" girl. Not only was she beautiful, but she was twenty-one. The perfect relationship (in my nineteen-year-old brain) to enable my binge drinking.

Until I turned twenty-one, this woman supplied me with all the alcohol I could ever hope for. Once I turned twenty-one, I was free to exercise my drinking muscles anytime I wanted. I became such a connoisseur that I took my talents behind the bar of a local restaurant, an experience that only served to fuel my love affair with heavy drinking.

These were the seeds planted in me in my early drinking career, and while it was fun, it also coincided with the fermentation of a darkness that had been dormant within me my entire life. That darkness was severe, debilitating anxiety. It was anxiety that dwarfed the worry and social anxieties that I had experienced as a child. I would soon long for the innocent worry and insecurity of childhood...That was amateur hour. Now I was entering the big leagues. While worry created clear disturbances on the Richter scale of anxiety, this new element was off the charts. I went from an eighteen-year-old who could maintain and suppress his depression and worry to a man crippled and cowering over the slightest fears.

My first panic attack came when I was twenty years old. I was studying for an organic chemistry exam, alone in my apartment, when this terrifying feeling of certainty came over me. Out of the blue, I became absolutely convinced that I was HIV positive. There was no rationale for this; there was zero evidence to support it. I was not promiscuous. I did not do any drugs that required injecting myself in any way, nor had I had a blood transfusion. Yet my brain screamed at me that I had the virus with such certainty that it caused me to self-destruct into a heap of paralyzing fear.

I couldn't move. I slumped down onto the floor and began sobbing for what seemed like hours. I had never experienced anything like it, and it came with absolutely no warning.

From an outside perspective, it may seem ludicrous to immediately, and without evidence, be convinced that I had a deadly autoimmune disease, but my brain formed this reality, and to me, at that very moment, it was as real as the floor upon which I was curled.

Why did I come to this conclusion? Because I had a sore throat and was tired.

I had read at one time that enlarged lymph nodes were one of the symptoms of HIV. Additionally, there is a feeling of fatigue and frequent sickness associated with the disease. For the first time in my life, my brain took an enormous jump from the rational to the improbable.

The feeling of fatigue could have been due to any number of causes. It could have been because I was overly stressed, smoking up to a pack of cigarettes a day, drinking heavily, a junk food enthusiast, or any combination of the above. I generally just didn't take care of myself, yet I believed with absolute certainty that my sore throat meant I was HIV positive.

I didn't know that what I was suffering from was a panic attack brought on by an anxiety disorder. I wouldn't know this for some time because I didn't know to ask about it, and the doctors I visited didn't know or care to ask about it.

When I went to get tested for HIV, the doctor asked the obvious questions.

"Are you sexually active?"

"Do you have multiple partners?"

"Do you use intravenous drugs?"

Upon answering no to all of them, the obvious follow-up question: "Then why the hell are you here?" never came up. I often wonder what would have happened if the doctor had dug just a little deeper. Would he have learned that a fantasized STD was not my problem, but rather a symptom of a psychological disorder? Despite the red flags, the doctor didn't make the connection. I went home from the clinic just as certain that I was HIV positive as when I had gone in and still none the wiser that this hypochondriacal episode was the result of an anxiety disorder.

After my test results came back negative, my immediate reaction was an enormous sense of relief, but that relief was short-lived. It created a void in which other fears could enter. Anxiety and panic manifested themselves in other ways. I felt as if the fear floated around inside of me, waiting for a single thing to latch on to and dominate my thoughts, and when it wrapped its claws around a concept, *BOOM!* I was down for the count.

I didn't know it at the time, but my anxiety was coupled with a highly obsessive personality. It was a dangerous combination. Anxiety, in the form of debilitating fear, focused itself on a single idea, and my attention fixated on that subject to the point of paralysis.

The HIV episode was my first experience with this obsessive anxiety. The next episode was cancer. I was certain I had Hodgkin's lymphoma (also centered around the fact that my lymph nodes seemed inflamed). Then when that fear was settled, it was another kind of cancer. Then appendicitis.

The list went on. If I saw a condition written in a book and it appeared very bad, I was convinced I had it. I was a full-blown hypochondriac, and despite the number of times I visited the medical clinic with crazy assumptions, the doctors never connected the dots.

Later, the obsessive hypochondria evolved into new avenues of fear. I feared that the police would come to arrest me. My excessive drinking resulted in more frequent blackouts by this time. Because I lost chunks of time, in times of sobriety, I thought I had certainly done something illegal while I was blacked out and that the police would surely be looking for me. Any rational human being in such a situation would not fear the police without cause, and if they did, they would probably put the bottle down for a while. However, alcohol continued to be my solution, and my solution was successful in immediately melting away the debilitating and irrational fears. The second I had a drink to my lips, my brain told me, "See? I told you it would be okay. You don't have a problem, and you have nothing to worry about." It was a cycle anchored in insanity.

The ridiculousness of this is not lost on me. I fully recognize that this was not rational thinking. Panic attacks and anxiety are irrational in nature. Unfortunately, those suffering from panic attacks do not believe they are being irrational. The fear can really be centered around anything: AIDS, cancer, the police, a stepfather, clowns, comets, dinosaurs...you name it. Anxiety induced in me irrational fears that appeared in every way to be very real.

Over time, I became more dependent on my solution. I immediately suppressed the fear by drinking. I still remember how my fears gradually slipped away with every sip. Life became a balance of drinking as much as I needed to calm my brain and convincing people that I didn't have a problem by projecting the appearance of sanity. It was a tightrope walk in a windstorm of denial.

At that time in my life, without any understanding of my problem, I failed to conduct a thorough examination of how I could resolve my anxiety in healthy ways. Instead, I chose to self-medicate with alcohol. As the drinking worsened, so, too, did the severity of the panic attacks and periods of paralyzing fear. It was around this time, about a year after my first panic attack, that I finally heard the term "generalized anxiety disorder." It sounded close to what I experienced on a daily basis. While other illnesses I tested for were irrational, this one made much more sense based on my symptoms. I knew that my fear was not normal, so I visited the clinic yet again with a different purpose in mind.

Maybe they could help me with my fear, I thought.

I told the doctor I was afraid all the time and worried about everything. After asking a series of questions, he prescribed me a medication called Paxil, and he said it helped treat generalized anxiety disorders.

That was the first time a name was given to my condition. Up until that point, I thought I was alone and crazy. I tried to hide it from everyone. The relief of discovering there was a name for my disorder was minimized by the realization that I would have to take medication to keep it at bay. What I didn't tell the doctor about was my propensity toward heavy drinking. I figured any mention of that would get me a finger wag at the very least and more likely a lecture on how I should probably just stop drinking to ease the anxiety. Of course, that would be the right first approach, but my dependence on my solution was anchored. One of my biggest fears at that moment was that I would be found out for what I really was: a hopeless drunk.

If that were to happen, I would risk never being able to drink again. It was as if the love of my life were at risk of being ripped from my hands. So, I kept my mouth shut about it, took the Paxil, and went on my way.

Paxil did little to ease my fears. The heavy alcohol consumption and anxiety while sober offset any benefit the medication would have offered. When I told the doctor that Paxil wasn't working, he offered other pharmaceutical solutions to me, including Wellbutrin and Xanax. Xanax did help with my anxiety, but the blackouts became substantially worse, so I chose to use it only in extreme circumstances. I don't really remember if the doctor who prescribed these medications recommended therapy, but even if he did, I was unlikely to take the advice. I did the math in my head and came to the conclusion that the first advice a therapist would give would be to stop drinking, which I was unwilling to do. I was too far down the road of dependency and a long way from understanding my real problems. I chose to continue poisoning myself and neglecting the right kind of help.

Oddly enough, despite all my attempts to medicate, illegal substances did not take for me. It wasn't from lack of trying, of course, but with the form of anxiety that I experienced, enhanced self-awareness is a byproduct. In my few experiences with marijuana, instead of a relaxing, stupefying experience, I experienced the exact opposite: paranoia and enhanced anxiety.

One such experience happened on a Saturday evening early in my freshman year of college. Some friends and I were hanging out in an apartment in Isla Vista. One young gentleman pulled out a three-foot bong. It was a magnificent contraption, a full yard of space for pot smoke to accumulate between the smoldering bud and the person about to get seriously fucked up. I mean, it took two people to operate the damn thing. I'm still not sure how the bong appeared halfway through the evening without us noticing it before or how the guy even brought it to the party without questions from the police who patrolled town. How does one hide such a conspicuous piece of equipment? On second thought, it's best not to answer that question.

A few people took turns taking hits off the giant glass wonder, a cartoonish endeavor given its size. I partook at one point and proceeded to feel my brain descend into a paradox of fog and heightened sensory awareness. This was probably my second time smoking marijuana, but the first time didn't really produce much of an effect on me. This one did.

I don't know how long into my high that we began watching television; it may have been minutes or hours. We turned on *Yellow Submarine*, the psychedelic Beatles cartoon, and began what would be a life-changing experience for me. Between the perplexing horror of weirdness that is *Yellow Submarine* and the yard's worth of THC molecules flowing through my system, I was, to put it mildly, tripping balls.

This was not a novice-level drug experience. This was "marijuana level: expert," and my brain was not equipped to handle it.

To top it off, my girlfriend, who didn't smoke pot, was with me and was giving me judgmental looks all night long. Her looks, in turn, caused me to judge myself. Now, I had two people judging me. I was in the throes of extreme paranoia. I continuously and mercilessly prodded at my girlfriend with "Are you all right?" She became increasingly annoyed and judgmental. Thus, we entered into a vicious cycle of judgment and paranoia that took me on a trip through marijuana hell for the remainder of the night.

Halfway through the movie, I decided enough was enough, and we left the party to go get something to eat—always a great idea when hardcore tripping on drugs.

My girlfriend joined me on my dazed adventure to the local burrito joint, mostly to ensure my safety and partially to continue judging me. I began scratching the top of my head incessantly. The scratching turned into an intense fear that I was digging my finger into my brain, but the itch just wouldn't go away. For some reason, this fear made me aware of my heartbeat, which seemed to be steadily increasing in rate and intensity.

I'm not sure if I finished my burrito, but we made our way back to my dorm room. My attention was still obsessively on my heart, which I was convinced was going to explode out of my chest and make a mess of my room. I opted to stare at the ceiling because everything else became too stimulating. That is how I would spend the next four hours until I somehow fell asleep.

In retrospect, this experience was likely one of the best things that has ever happened to me because it gave me self-realization. I recognized that if marijuana had this effect on me, I didn't want to know what cocaine, acid, heroin, or other substances would do to me. So, I simply never tried them, mainly out of fear—one of the few times that fear saved my life—and partially because I had already found a solution with alcohol.

Alcohol didn't make me paranoid, at least until I sobered up. Alcohol immediately quieted the monster in my brain. It was no longer just a solution for my social awkwardness. Unlike pot, it was now a solution to calm my mind when it was acting against me. Unfortunately, it wasn't the solution to everything. My anxiety and alcohol dependence worked together to ruin my grades. I began to lose control, and I was more hostile with the people close to me. The hangovers and sickness I managed to avoid in the past started becoming a thing for me. This meant I had to try much harder to hide my condition and lie more to myself about the control I didn't have. Of course, it never worked. I started hating who I was and where I was presently, and I began fixating on the future.

"It will get better when I finish school," I told myself, along with other promises about the future. I knew changing my habits would require tremendous change within me, and I wasn't ready to make those changes. I feared what my brain might put me through without alcohol as a silencer. So, I blamed my current circumstances and promised it would be different in the future. The cycle was the very definition of insanity.

My belief that things would improve with a change in surroundings and circumstance led me to leave Santa Barbara shortly after graduating from UCSB. Perhaps it is ironic that I graduated with a degree in psychology but failed to grasp the problems with my own mind. Maybe the professors ignored it, or maybe it was just selective attention on my part, but I don't remember any of the courses addressing anxiety, depression, or substance abuse. I do remember a lot of discussion related to extreme and rare case studies, brain injury, and psychopathic behavior, all of which are sexy topics of conversation for the psychology enthusiast.

The situational change I decided to make was to join the corporate workforce in the relatively safe surroundings of my family's business. My girlfriend, Marie, and I moved to Orange County, and I began work in our Research and Development department. Shortly thereafter, I married Marie, and we attempted to build a normal, cookie-cutter life.

I hoped that the move back to the familiar surroundings of my childhood would wipe clean the psychological turmoil I had experienced in college. In fact, I even attempted to quit drinking as a fresh start, but that, of course, was short-lived. It became apparent very quickly that a change in geography was not the key to curbing my excessive drinking.

The problem was not the surroundings; the problem was me. I carried that internal turmoil with me wherever I went, and I numbed the pain with alcohol. I justified it all because I was still able to function within the society around me. It was a living hell that I was able to hide through tremendous effort. Despite my fear and frequent drunkenness, I maintained my composure enough throughout the course of the day to do my job effectively, pay our bills, and give little indication of my problems. I was the very definition of a "functional alcoholic," which is an oxymoron because it's just a charade. Within a culture where alcohol is plentiful and drinking is legal and often encouraged, people with an alcohol problem tend to hide it in plain sight until a major alcoholic event occurs. Even then, many alcoholics, and even their loved ones, will overlook or dismiss the incident as a one-off or an out-of-character event because, well, "He's usually such a good guy" or "He doesn't fit the picture of an alcoholic." That may be true based on appearances, but he also has a disease, one that he is trying desperately to cover up while living in constant fear of being discovered and battling his own demons.

Those who have experienced it know alcoholism is not always as blatant as it is depicted in our culture. It is not all dumpster diving and passing out in the streets. In most cases, alcoholics are living and working, often productively, within society, trying desperately to maintain the appearance of normalcy and "control" their substance abuse. The farce has an expiration date, and the truth eventually comes out. Alcoholism is what's called a "progressive" disease—one that starts out very subtly and gradually becomes something much darker.

Although I felt like I was leaving the darkness behind me, it was still ahead of me. I continued to live a seemingly normal life. I tried desperately to model my parents' lifestyle. They always seemed to live blissfully, without any worries. I craved that. I imagined a life without anxiety or alcohol dependency and tried everything I could to suppress my fear, anxiety, and depression. Everything, that is, except giving up drinking.

After some time, Marie and I started having children. First, we had Sarah in 2007, and then we had Zachary in 2011. I hoped that having children would change me into a better human being, but I continued to feel broken and fearful. The only difference was my commitments kept growing in scale and importance. Fatherhood created an even deeper sense of shame around the fact that I could not change.

I was no longer a single man whose choices only affected himself. I was responsible for a family. Even then I denied I had a problem *because* I was able to function as a father and husband. In addition to being a social lubricant and medication for anxiety, drinking became a way to make myself feel "happier." It had that effect for a while, but as drinking made me happier, it also made sobriety less pleasant. Then the anxiety kicked in, and my relationships suffered. Alcohol became a necessity. I needed it to function so I could live without the fear and suppress my unhappiness. After all, if I wasn't happy, how could I be any good to my family?

This is one of the natural progressions of alcoholism. It is often said, and I find it to be true in my own experience, that drinking is at first fun, then it's fun with problems, and then it's just problems.

I was chasing a feeling that alcohol could never give me again. Whether or not the anxiety led to the drinking or the drinking led to the anxiety is a "chicken and egg" argument, and it didn't really matter. What mattered was that I was broken. My spiritual health, my mental health, my physical health, and my perspective were all broken.

During the early years of my new family, I created a set of rules all designed to convince myself that I didn't have a drinking problem. It was not dissimilar to the rules in the movie *Gremlins* on how to take care of a Mogwai. Breaking them, I felt, would increase the chances of me turning into an ugly, chaotic gremlin.

1. Do not drink more than one bottle of wine in one sitting. (This one was often broken very quickly.)
2. Do not drink before five in the afternoon.
3. Do not drink on a work night. Only drink on the weekends. (The weekends would gradually begin to include Sunday night, Thursday night, and sometimes Monday night.)
4. Do not drink hard alcohol. Stick to beer and wine.
5. Never drink and drive.

While I frequently broke my rules, as long as I held on to one of them, I convinced myself that I didn't have a problem. It was easy for me to justify my drinking because of the things I didn't do rather than acknowledge the destructive nature of my drinking because of the things that I did do. I was never violent; I didn't hide bottles under the bed; I stayed away from hard alcohol; I was able to stay "sober" a few days out of the week (as miserable as it was to do so); and never, ever, did I drink and drive.

Drinking and driving was simply a line I would not cross for over a decade of drinking. I vehemently hated people who drank and drove. They risked the lives of innocent people, which was absolutely abhorrent to me. Even if I did get out-of-control drunk, I never sank to that level of inhumanity.

Until I did.

Transition

IRONMAN TEXAS, 2015. MILE 2.4.

"Holy crap, I made it!"

I still had 138.2 miles to go, but I felt like a champion as I took to my amphibious assault on The Woodlands, a township just a short drive north of Houston, Texas. Moments earlier, the murky, dark infinity of the lake below me showed no signs of a bottom. It was enough to send my mind racing, considering all that could be below me: snakes, mutants, WMDs, and competitors from previous years' races who had been absorbed by the lake floor to be eternally digested, like an aquatic Sarlacc. Yeah, staring blankly at a murky abyss for over an hour can lead to a few hallucinations.

As I approached the swim finish, I lifted my head for every stroke to see the cheers and bells of the spectators interrupt the relative peace of the underwater world. It was like the opening scene of *Saving Private Ryan*, minus the bullets and death and with a lot more neoprene and Body Glide.

As I reached the end of the swim, one hand grasped the stair rail, and the other was grasped by a volunteer in a bright orange shirt. He yanked me up as if I were a toddler, a feat made all the more impressive by the fact that he had to have been older than seventy.

This jolt onto the shore was my cue to start running. As I did, I felt my heart try urgently to supply much-needed blood to my legs, the extremities that I had been neglecting for the past hour and twenty minutes. I more than made up for the neglect over the next nine hours of nonstop work. The shock of abrupt and violent movement caused instant cramping in my legs, which forced me to walk a few steps while the blood supply caught up. Trudging down the path to Transition 1, or T1, I awkwardly unzipped my speedsuit (which didn't live up to its name this day) and peeled it down to my waist.

I grabbed a couple cups of water and spilled them over my head, hoping to look like I knew what I was doing. I didn't.

"Four-six-one!" a man shouted into a blowhorn as I ran past. It took me a second to realize that was my race number. A moment later, a big blue bag was shoved into my chest by a volunteer. This bag contained my bike gear: helmet, shoes, nutrition, and the rest of the equipment that would assist me through the next 112 miles. I ripped it open as another volunteer guided me into a big white tent.

The men's changing tent at an Ironman event is like a gym locker room on steroids. It was tan lines galore as men rushed to change from their swimwear to their bike gear. Others were just clamoring to get through and onto their bikes. The smell inside the tent was intensified by the heat and humidity. I imagine it was similar to what a long-abandoned cheese factory would smell like if it was left mid-Limburger production. My elevated heart rate and adrenaline, mixed with the flurry of activity and sheer volume of naked bodies, made it difficult to stay focused on the task at hand.

The transition, in theory, seems pretty simple. All I had to do was take off my speedsuit, put on my bike shoes and helmet, place my speedsuit and goggles into the blue bag, grab my nutrition and sunglasses, and go. In practice, however, with my heart rate somewhere around 170 beats per minute and the heat index inside the tent at around 110 degrees, I ended up just staring blankly at my ripped blue bag for what seemed like five minutes.

Finally, another man in an orange shirt came by to help me.

"Hand me your speedsuit," he instructed.

It's amazing how a simple instruction can snap one back into focus. I obliged and he handed me my helmet. I managed to put it on, followed by my shoes.

The man handed me my glasses, my bag full of salt tablets, and a canister of Vaseline. I apologized profusely as I grabbed a handful of the warm jelly and shoved it down my pants, creepily rubbing it into my nether regions as the volunteer looked on, intrigued and disgusted. It was an intimate moment that both of us would hope to forget, but it would surely be burned into our memories. Such is the ugliness that occurs in the Ironman changing tent. Much like Las Vegas, what happens in the changing tent stays in the changing tent.

I ran out into the fresh air, awkwardly tiptoeing in my cleats over the muddy grass. I emerged and turned down the first aisle of bikes and came to find my trusted steed, hanging right where I had left her a little over an hour before. The solid black beauty was about to carry me as I rode a single loop around the middle of Texas, a mostly flat, mostly rural area of the state where they do everything bigger, including hating cyclists.

I ran with my bike up to the "bike mount" area, where I clumsily climbed onto my bike and clipped my shoes into the pedals. Off I rode into the wilderness, where I spent nearly five hours cranking away.

3

RECOVERY

I came out of my blackout in the back of a police car. There was a combination of intense shame and confusion. Confusion because I didn't know what was happening. Shame because I knew *exactly* what was happening.

I looked out the window of the squad car to discover a familiar setting: my house, my street, and my neighbors staring. Yet there were unfamiliar and horrific scenes also: a number of police cars and policemen, my wife sobbing on the curb, and my totaled car.

In most cases, coming out of a blackout would cause me extreme anxiety. I was forced to try to reassemble the pieces of the night before, hoping that I hadn't embarrassed myself too badly, all while trying to calm an ever-increasing fear that I didn't know. In many cases, the anxiety was unwarranted. Most times, I simply got drunk off my ass, spent the evening alone and embarrassing only myself, before eventually passing out. The anxiety of coming out of a blackout would so overwhelm me that I would often begin numbing the pain with alcohol first thing in the morning.

In this particular instance, based on the scene unfolding around me, it was clear I had reason to be fearful, but it wasn't the debilitating fear I had experienced so many times before that overwhelmed me. This wasn't some surreal situation made up in my anxious brain; this was real. Fear had done its job. Now I felt a deep, dark, and well-justified shame and depression.

I tried to remember how I had ended up in the back of a police car, but I just couldn't recall the circumstances sur- rounding my present situation. I later pieced together that I was likely still drunk from the night before when I woke up, drank more in the early morning before I went surfing, and then drank more after surfing. On my way home, I ran a red light before turning into my neighborhood and crashing into another car. Thank God nobody was injured.

As my neighbors looked on, I proceeded to fail the field sobriety tests given to me, a humiliating formality considering my state. The police finished their investigation and drove me to the Orange County jail where I spent the evening contem- plating my fate and planning my escape from life.

If it weren't obvious before, it was now clear that nobody was safe from me. I wasn't the only one suffering. I was causing oth- ers to suffer as well. In my mind, I was not fit to be a part of this world anymore. I only caused harm and presented a significant danger to those around me, something I desperately did not want to be. I desired so much to be a compassionate, loving, and harmless individual, but my actions produced the exact opposite results—selfishness, pain, and wreckage. I could no longer control myself, and it was getting to the point that I could possibly kill someone. My solution was no longer working. It hadn't been for a very long time, but I couldn't admit it until it was too late. Now, there was no solution left for me to use. The only option now was to remove myself from this Earth, for the benefit of my family and the rest of humanity. For the first time in my life, I thought about killing myself.

I had always been afraid of dying. The uncertainty and the eternity of what lay beyond this life was terrifying to me. Plus, I had such a low opinion of myself that I figured that any beautiful afterlife that existed wouldn't want me, so why on earth would I want to speed up the process? I was scared of living, but the fear of death had always overwhelmed it. Until now. Now I had no fear of death. Just shame.

Suicide came to me not as a means of escaping my earthly fate, but more as a means to remove myself as a concern. I was a burden in this world, and I caused my family and most other people more pain than pleasure. It would be a mercy to them, not me—or at least that's the way I saw it. I didn't want to live this way, and I thought that surely nobody else wanted me around either.

It will come as no surprise that jail is not a pleasant place. Upon my arrival, I received a bologna sandwich, the highlight of the next twenty-four hours. The rest of the time was spent sitting alone, battling claustrophobia and dark thoughts between intermittent belittling from the guards. I wasn't as affected by that as I was by the internal monologue that consumed my thoughts. The voice in my head incessantly called me a worthless piece of shit and told me to just kill myself. The anxiety and shame I felt was overwhelming. I was no longer battling irrational fear; this was legitimate. I was facing the serious consequences of my actions. *What is to become of me? What happened to the other party involved in the crash? How is my family reacting to this?*

Out of all the senses, it was the smell I remember the most. I recall the putrid smell of my body, still rancid from wearing a soaking wetsuit for many hours. But I can most easily conjure the smell of alcohol on my breath that served as a brutal reminder of my complete lack of control over it and my life.

I had tried on a few occasions to get sober. Each time, I ended up drunk again. It's clear now that my motive for sobriety in the past was only to appease my family after a particularly bad night. After a few sober weeks, I convinced myself, and my family, that I could start drinking again and this time keep it under control. It never worked out that way. Inevitably, my drinking always got worse. The blackouts became more frequent; I caused more damage, and I experienced more shame. This time around, I was a danger to others.

After my stay in jail, I was processed out and shuffled off into the middle of the night. Unsurprisingly, there were no well-wishes from the jail staff as I exited. As I walked along the yellow line painted onto the cold concrete floor, young officers relentlessly mocked my fellow inmates and me.

"We'll probably be seeing you again tomorrow...and the next day, you fucking drunk," said one officer.

It hurt, but I couldn't blame him for saying that. He saw people at their worst on a daily basis. I couldn't begin to imagine the frustration that would cause. Certainly, it would be easy to become jaded and lash out at people who were at their worst. After all, I was telling myself the same story.

The insult forced me to reflect on my own hopelessness. The paths before me were now clear: death or incarceration. These were the choices I had.

Choice.

A revelation occurred to me as I thought about these two options. My path was a choice. As helpless as I felt at the time, I began to recognize that my failure at managing my own life was the result of my attempts to control it. The reality was that I couldn't manage something I didn't control.

If this was a choice, surely there could be a third option. If the current path led to death or incarceration, there must be an alternative path. Then it came to me. While my previous attempts at sobriety were not successful, something from those first experiences in recovery stuck in my brain. I couldn't do it on my own because I lost control. I needed to surrender control over my life because, after all, I already had. I had surrendered to alcohol and anxiety as my higher powers a long time ago. I needed a higher power that could allow me to overcome the addiction and the fear. If I wanted to live, and get sober, I needed to be all in on my recovery.

I needed help, and for the first time in my life, I was willing to give up control over my own life to get it.

———◆———

"Wait a year before making any major life changes." People with long stretches of sobriety always advise newcomers to avoid any major distractions while getting sober. Early sobriety demands structure, routine, and accountability. Every single day: eat, sleep, go to meetings, work the steps, and repeat.

"Sobriety should be number one. Before work, before family, before everything."

These warnings were ominous, often delivered in a somber tone as if the "old-timers" had seen the disastrous effects of others not heeding the advice a million times. I had been one of those millions. Previously, the level of commitment and discipline required to follow this very simple advice was always a bit much for me.

Before family? *Really?* So, if a family member is dying, I need to be in meetings before spending time with that loved one?

Yes.

I always had trouble with that concept. It never seemed like the moral thing to do. I thought it was selfish to go to Alcoholics Anonymous meetings every day or work with a sponsor as a priority over family or work. I never prioritized sobriety in my life because it just didn't ever feel that desperate, and when I perceived the demand for commitment was becoming too overwhelming, I stopped working a program and ultimately failed.

It wasn't that my family or work demanded all of my time. Even though I had a demanding job (I was now well entrenched in the family business), a wife, and two young children, I fooled myself with the belief that I didn't have time to commit to sobriety. More accurately, I needed an excuse. I was not willing to give up the false sense of control I had over my drinking. My selfishness and ego actually prevented me from the vulnerability necessary to surrender to a daily life of sobriety.

The lack of commitment in these early attempts at sobriety resulted in a gradual, but not unexpected, descent back into the depths of active alcoholism every single time. It is a common theme, sadly one that is shared by many alcoholics and addicts. While we may come into recovery with a 90 percent commitment to get and stay clean, the remaining 10 percent will take us back out. One moment of weakness is powerful and pervasive. It's a cancer. All it takes is one slip. Once we drink, we are right back to our old habits.

My previous attempts at sobriety were borne of similar circumstances. I would do something foolish while drunk and embarrassed myself or my wife. The next morning, while in a hungover haze of humiliation, anxiety, and shame, I resolved to quit drinking and start going to AA meetings—often at the insistence of my wife and family. While the shame and guilt were still with me, I attended some AA meetings and began feeling good about myself again. Sobriety began to feel comfortable after some time, and I started to enjoy life without alcohol. As I met more people in recovery, things started getting a little too "real" for me. This became especially true when I faced the uncomfortable question presented by members of AA with long-term sobriety. "Do you have a sponsor?"

It was if they asked me if I would listen to their pyramid scheme pitch while standing naked in the men's locker room. It was an awkward conversation I didn't want to have. I was going to say no, and I knew that I would have to dodge the fact that I believed it was a crackpot idea.

I didn't *really* think it was a crackpot idea. I witnessed many people succeeding in sobriety by working the steps with a sponsor. In the back of my mind, however, finding a sponsor meant closing the door on an AA exit strategy. If I avoided the meaningful personal and emotional ties to the program, it would be easy to quietly fade away if I needed to. This truth may have been veiled by superficial beliefs that I just didn't have time to work the steps or that I couldn't find a sponsor who I could relate to, but in reality, jumping into recovery led to an irrational fear of sobriety.

So, this is really it. I'm never *drinking again,* was my way of thinking.

As soon as this thought crept into my sober mind, the door to relapse cracked open. The deeper I journeyed into recovery, the stronger my relationships with sober people became, and the more accountable I became to staying sober, the more the reality sank in that I could never drink again. The certainty and finality of this belief was a powder keg that would eventually explode in epic fashion.

As long as I had only one foot in the door of sobriety, it was still possible in my broken and self-centered mindset to justify a drink. Regardless of how many hands were trying to pull me deeper into recovery, one foot out was always a stronger force. Despite the fact that I *thought* I was getting a lot from recovery, and I thought my sobriety was bulletproof, I couldn't accept the finality of sobriety.

What if I became overwhelmed with anxiety? How would I cope in social situations where alcohol was present? I would surely become a pariah if I was unable to drink. The reality was that living a life where alcohol was a primary theme was all I ever knew in my adult life. It had always been there, and because of that, I didn't really know how to live without it. I would have to face all of my fears, insecurities, anger, and unhappiness *sober*. I couldn't embrace the idea of never drinking again. *Never* was a scary word. Thus, keeping the door open to a drink was oddly comforting. A plan to drink was always brewing in my subconscious.

Such was the case in one of my early attempts at sobriety in 2006. It began one morning as I came to, as if awakening from a coma. I didn't remember the night before, but the anger, sadness, and demoralization on my wife's face told the story. The ultimatum was given: either go to AA to get sober or lose my wife. Afraid to lose my wife, I chose AA.

I went to meetings about once a week for a few months, generally keeping my distance from members of the group, lest I get sucked in to their little cult. Gradually, after just a few short months of recovery, I stopped going to meetings. I told my wife that I couldn't relate to anyone there; unlike them, I had my shit together. I could stay sober on my own.

I did...for a while. Without a program, I didn't have the tools to manage my emotions. Anxiety, anger, and resentment overtook me. Anger is a manifestation of fear, and since I had done nothing to address my fears and resentments, they would begin to consume me. Even though I wasn't a social drinker, I would begin to feel annoyed in social situations where other people were drinking, and I wasn't able to share in their "enjoyment." I liked to drink alone. My mind would do everything it could to manipulate my way to a drink.

The tipping point (the point where I "tipped" a drink into my mouth) came on the Big Island of Hawaii in September 2006. I was about nine months sober at the time, but I hadn't been to a recovery program in many months. My wife and I were on vacation, at a restaurant at the Royal Kona Hotel. As we sat there in this beautiful setting overlooking Kailua Bay, I made a conscious decision to end my sobriety.

Unbeknownst to me at the time, I was sitting only a few hundred meters away from the starting line of one of the most iconic celebrations on the planet. Every year, thousands of the fittest people in the world descend upon Kona to participate in the Ironman World Championship. A few go to compete. Most are there to celebrate the amazing achievement of having qualified for the Super Bowl of triathlons. These are the very best in the world, and many of them have overcome significant challenges to be one of those few.

While I had seen this race on television in the past and was in awe of the enormity of it, it was the farthest thing from my mind at that moment. Everything was. Only one thing was on my mind: how to convince my wife that I was entitled to begin drinking again.

It was a plan many months in the making. I began to provide verbal evidence that I was cured and should be allowed to have a Mai Tai in Hawaii. I had been sober for months without a program. Surely, I no longer had a problem and could drink normally again. It had been long enough. After all, we were on vacation.

I played the guilt card. The unspoken ultimatum that if I couldn't have a drink while on vacation, I would be an insufferable, passive-aggressive prick. I was holding my own wife hostage so that I could destroy nine months of sobriety and binge drink my way through the Hawaiian Islands. I didn't need her permission to drink, of course. But her permission would validate my own warped opinion. She could be my partner in crime. My enabler.

Of course, she complied, mostly out of exhaustion rather than agreement, and I proceeded to relapse back into alcoholic oblivion. In the same place where thousands of athletes started a 140.6-mile journey through the lava fields to achieve

something incredible and celebrate the act of living, I was starting a journey into five more years through hell. Five more years
of obsessive and excessive drinking. Five more years of anxiety,
depression, loss of control, and hopelessness.

I never figured out a way to drink like a normal person. The
truth is that I never even *wanted* to drink like a normal person.
I didn't come to that realization until I got sober. The idea of
just having "a drink or two" doesn't appeal to me. The obsessive
nature of my mind leads me to think of drinking compulsively
to inebriation and beyond. Even now, I could never simply
think of a single drink. My mind automatically goes to the bottle, or bottles—enough so that I cannot physically drink more.

If, for any reason, I ran out of alcohol or was unable to continue drinking, I was consumed with grief. The only thing to
which I can equate it is the feeling of being dumped by a true love.

Regardless of how long I had been sober, all it took was a
single sip and the cycle of misery started again. Before too
long, I once again drank myself into a blackout, breaking the
rules I had set for myself, embarrassing myself and my wife,
and hiding empty bottles until the guilt and shame became
too much to bear.

Then came the crash and the DUI. It was my rock bottom. It
was an event so frightening and damaging that it caused me to
question whether I deserve to live. I had broken my very last
rule and put people in danger. I turned into someone I hated
and who was hated by society. Only sheer luck kept me from
killing or injuring anyone else.

It opened a door that, up to that point, had never been opened. The door to willingness. With willingness came an open mind to the advice that the old-timers had given me time and again.

"Sobriety should be number one."

"Wait a year before making any life changes."

Walking out of the jail cell, sobriety became number one.

When I walked into my first AA meeting after the crash, I walked in with both feet. I left nothing behind outside the doors. I had nothing. This was the last option I had and the last house on the block that would have me, and I gave myself to it fully. I transcended guilt and shame as the primary reasons to get sober. After all, they were often my reasons for getting drunk. It was not enough for me to *need* sobriety. I had to *want* it more than anything else in my life, including my family, my job...

Everything.

Full immersion meant daily AA meetings, saying yes to invitations from other recovering alcoholics to coffee or breakfast meetings, and constant contact with sober people. I had to hang on to sobriety like my life depended on it because it did. If I drank again, the only outcome would be death or incarceration. It took a drunk driving accident to bring me into the rooms this time. If I couldn't be saved now, I would be lost. There was always a lower bottom, and I didn't want to find out what that was.

This attitude made a big difference during this round of sobriety. Instead of wanting to leave and find another drink, I wanted desperately to stay. If I could avoid taking the first drink, there may be hope.

Hope.

Hope was a concept that I could not wrap my head around. Yet, I prayed for help while still in a half-drunken stupor in the Orange County jail. During those prayers, I began to feel as though there was a glimmer of hope. I remembered all the trite sayings sober people had repeated in the past.

"It works if you work it."

"Don't leave before the miracle happens."

"Keep coming back."

As I sat in an AA meeting, completely broken, lost, and uncertain of my freedom in the near future, I felt a peace I had never felt before because I could finally acknowledge who I really was and work toward a solution.

I spent those early days in recovery listening to the experiences of sober people, and hope began to grow. I opened my heart and mind to sobriety and began to do the work necessary to embrace recovery; I began to feel like I was no longer hopeless.

The fresh wound of a traumatic event can be enough to spark the willingness and humility to accept help, but as that wound begins to heal, the pain that triggered that willingness becomes a distant memory. Without continued immersion and accountability within the community of sobriety, the willingness may fade. I knew based on my experience that the chance of a relapse was a very real probability for me if I didn't hold on to that willingness with all my might, so I immediately immersed myself within the community, fully and without hesitation. If a DUI accident was not enough to give me the sustained willingness to maintain sobriety, nothing would.

Practicing the advice of others and finding community in other people who shared my malady helped me find some relief from my anxiety. Despite the uphill legal battle I had yet to face, panic and fear no longer debilitated me. As long as I got my ass to meetings, I was able to face whatever road was ahead of me. I could finally accept my circumstances, focus on what I could control, and quell the fear of what might happen in the future. Yes, I was facing possible jail time, but at that very moment, I was sober, and I was working on becoming a better human being. The consequences would be what they were. I could not change the past, but I could change the person I would become.

In the early days and months of my sobriety, many people stood out to me as successful in sobriety. They weren't successful because they made a lot of money or were high-powered businesspeople. It wasn't necessarily their family lives or their charm. In fact, what attracted me most to the successful people in AA was their attitude toward life. Ultimately, it was their response to imperfection. Many of these people were just scraping by financially: they were divorced; they had children in jail; they had chronic diseases. They had every excuse to be miserable, angry, and resentful, but one thing stood out to me about all of these people.

They were happy.

How could people with alcoholism, living in a prison of sobriety with deep personal problems, be happy? This was a question I could not answer, but I wanted to find out. I wanted what these people had: unwavering joy, gratitude, and grace.

Jim personified this attitude, and I very quickly gravitated toward him as an example of what I wanted to become. Well over two decades sober, seemingly nothing ever got to him. Many of the people in AA vented in anger during a share, sighed in boredom during the readings, or showed at least a glimmer of evidence that their serenity was compromised, but not Jim. Jim was always grateful and always wise, and people listened when he spoke.

I wanted what Jim had.

But I was afraid. Despite his kind demeanor and constant willingness to reach out to me, I feared both the inevitable rejection and the commitment that would result from asking him to be my sponsor. Fear was the enemy, and to overcome the fear, I had to get out of my head. I had to do what was called in AA "opposite action." Instead of retreating, I leaned in.

I was sitting in a parking lot outside of my court-appointed DUI class, staring at Jim's phone number on a wrinkled piece of paper. My palms were sweaty, and I was practicing the conversation I would have with Jim in my head. I snapped out of this for a second and realized that I felt like a teenage boy nervously asking a girl to the prom.

"This is silly," I said. "Just do it already. Your life depends on it!"

I dialed the phone, and Jim picked up.

"Adam," the voice on the other end of the line said.

I wasn't expecting him to say my name. I had forgotten that when we exchanged numbers, he programmed my number into his phone.

"Hi, Jim. This is Adam from the meeting," I said sheepishly, as if it were rehearsed, and I hadn't heard him just say my name. It was, and I did.

After a perfectly awkward silence that I'm sure Jim allowed to persist for his own amusement, I continued, "I was wondering if, um, you would be my sponsor?"

Jim didn't hesitate. "Absolutely, but there's a condition..."

Uh oh, I thought. *Here it comes.* I knew there would be a condition. What would it be? Would I need to wash his car every weekend or do his landscaping? Would I be like Daniel-san to his Mr. Miyagi? Or would I just be hazed in some weird AA fraternity sort of way? I felt apprehension kick in immediately.

He continued, "Sobriety isn't something you *need*. You have to *want* it more than anything else in the world. More than your job, more than your family, more than anything."

"I do want it," I said, almost defensively. Then I caught myself and repeated the phrase as a statement of fact. "I *do* want it, more than anything else."

"Good," he said. "I'll see you tomorrow when we'll work on step one. Bring your Big Book."

The Heat

IRONMAN LOS CABOS, 2014. MILE 74.

Cresting one of the many hills on the bike course, I caught a view of the deep blue ocean. The iconic arches of Cabo San Lucas sprawled out into the sea on the horizon, like a medieval depiction of a sea serpent slipping in and out of the water.

At that moment, all I could think about was how much I wanted to get back into that water, the same water I had been eager to exit a few short hours earlier. I wanted to wash off the sweat and soak my aching muscles. I desired to lay back, float, and let the gentle waves sway my body back and forth.

I shook away the thought and went back to the task at hand, which was to continue pushing the pedals and accelerate down yet another hill, building momentum that would hopefully carry me up to the crest of the next. It was hot and windy now, and the crosswind only served to blow hot, dry air sideways into my deep-rimmed wheels. Every gust pushed my bike toward the shoulder, and I had to use valuable energy to fight it back onto the road.

The bike course ping-ponged between the two towns that make up Los Cabos—Cabo San Lucas and San Jose del Cabo. Ultimately, we would finish the three laps of the bike course in the Northeast town of San Jose del Cabo, where we started our run and would (hopefully) finish the race. But that was still a long way off.

The sweat, which was pouring from my forehead earlier in the race, now seemed nonexistent. I struggled to stay cool and hydrated. Aid stations were spread out about every fifteen miles, which was just enough time for me to finish off my last bottle, discard it, and replace it with a full one. Despite this, I felt like I could not take in enough water to stave off dehydration.

I needed to stop worrying and get out of my head. Just stick to the plan: finish a bottle between every aid station. Any more wouldn't help me stay hydrated; it would only sit in my stomach and slosh around until I either puked it out or worse.

Salt was my friend. I consumed sports drinks constantly to keep a steady supply in my body to avoid hyponatremia. As long as I stopped questioning my nutrition and hydration plan and stuck to it, I would be fine. After all, I had practiced it over and over again in training. Ritual, routine, consistency, discipline...these were all elements that dramatically elevated my chances of success in a race. The simple action of taking a sip of nutrition every fifteen minutes, followed by a swig of water, was something I could control, and staying disciplined with that simple action would make a tremendous difference in how the things I couldn't control— like weather, mechanical issues, or other race conditions— affected me. They were lessons I learned from sobriety.

"Control the controllables," my coach told me. My AA sponsor always told me the same. It was advice taken directly from the serenity prayer. "Grant me the serenity to accept the things I cannot change, the courage to change the things I can, and the wisdom to know the difference."

My watch beeped. Another fifteen minutes had passed, and it was time to take another sip of my concentrated sports drink. I sat up from the aerobars, stretched my back, and grabbed my bottle to take a quick swig, immediately followed by a big gulp of plain water from another bottle. The result, ideally, was a diluted solution of pure sugar and electrolytes to fuel me for the next fifteen minutes.

The drink itself tasted like the concentrated syrup for lemon-lime soda, without the carbonation and extra water. Just the pure sugary goodness that an eight-year-old would only dream of. It was a mixture of maltodextrin and sucrose, which would break down and metabolize into glucose. I had to wash each sip down with a big gulp of water to increase the dilution as the drink went into my stomach. Too high a concentration of carbohydrates would cause gastrointestinal issues. So far, it was working, and I was avoiding the GI issues, but I still had a lot of race left to go, including a full marathon.

Taking sips of the drink every fifteen minutes helped me to pass the time. One hundred twelve miles is a long time to be on a bike, and as crazy as it sounds, the simple act of counting down to the next intake of calories gave me something to look forward to.

My pace began to slow as the grade of the climb increased and the breeze faded. I pressed on, climbing through the heat of the midday sun, knowing that once I crested the hill that I would once again be greeted with more wind. That wind was a blessing and a curse. I wanted it desperately when it wasn't there, but when it was, it forced me to work harder to control the bike.

As I reached the turnaround at Cabo San Lucas and began the haul back to San Jose del Cabo, I sighed. "One and a half more loops to go."

I caught myself and remembered to focus on the present. The rest of the race would come later. I focused on what I could control in the present.

4

ANXIETY
SUPERHERO

Sobriety not only required abstinence from alcohol, but it also required a complete transformation of my thoughts and behaviors. If I didn't change the person I was, I would either end up a miserable wreck, a drunk, or both. Sobriety was not just the condition of not drinking; it was a spiritual, mental, and physical adaptation to a new way of living. My alcoholism was rooted deeply in an obsession for control, resentment, fear, and an intense anxiety disorder. Simply quitting drinking does not automatically alleviate those issues. In fact, those issues are the primary part of the "-ism" in alcoholism.

AA did much to help me face these issues head on. It forced me to complete a fourth-step inventory. After completing the first three of twelve steps in arduous detail at the recommendation and oversight of my sponsor, Jim, I stared down the barrel of the fourth step: "Make a searching and fearless moral inventory of ourselves."

A searching and fearless moral inventory. Never had so few words presented so succinctly what caused me so much discomfort. First of all, I wasn't fearless. I had spent my whole life fear*ful*. How could I possibly be fearless? It seemed like a paradox to me. Second, I didn't believe I was moral. I spent the last decade or more of my life hiding my true self from people and behaving like a self-centered wrecking ball.

Whereas the first three steps are mostly philosophical in nature (admitting we're alcoholics and that a higher power must be sought for serenity and spiritual awakening), step four is where the rubber hits the road. It's where a lot of alcoholics fall out of the program. It's the point at which I needed to turn my attention inward and face myself truthfully, to face the person I really was, to search deep for defects of character, and to admit, on paper, my darkest secrets. It was a purge of everything, and it was really fucking hard.

Let me be clear: the act of putting pen to paper is not difficult. Deep down, I knew what was wrong, just as every defeated alcoholic does. The hard part is facing the darkest part of ourselves in rigorous detail. It's jumping head-first into an ice-cold bath of reality, one that we drank to avoid for years, and sometimes decades. The inventory forces us to address root causes, not just superficial baloney. Additionally, we address the entrenched ego. This is the part of ourselves that tells us that we are right and others are wrong—the part that holds a grudge and can't forgive, and the part that tells us that we can make it on our own.

In my previous experience with sobriety, I left as soon as it was time for me to complete the fourth step. This time, I was willing to be honest and overcome my fear because the alternative seemed far more frightening.

Jim made the process as effective and achievable as possible by outlining a simple plan. We completed the fourth step over a period of a few weeks, making sure I was as rigorous and thorough as possible. For the first week, he provided me a crudely drawn grid of paper with a word written in all caps at the top. That word was "RESENTMENTS."

Within the worksheet, I was asked to specifically lay out what I was angry at—whether it be people, situations, or anything that caused resentment—and then lay out what part of me felt hurt. This part was easy. I could go on for days about who wronged me and how it affected me. I was a pity-party expert. It was the next few columns that were challenging to me.

The next column asked: Where was I to blame?

How could I possibly be blamed if I were the victim? I struggled with this until Jim simplified it for me by explaining that it all comes back to the things we can and can't control. We can't control how people treat us, but we can control our reactions to that treatment. Being imperfect beings, we rarely react to mistreatment with grace. We should strive to treat others with the same amount of grace as we would hope to be given.

With this explanation, it was easier to find my responsibility in every situation and acknowledge it. One thing I found by doing this was that I was very resentful that I allowed myself to drive drunk and put another person's life in danger. I was not only ashamed but angry. I hated that I not only let myself down but let others down as well. The process of doing an inventory on resentments gave me the vulnerability to forgive and make peace with myself.

A similar grid was handed to me the following week with the word "FEARS" written along the top. Just seeing the word triggered the feeling. *How could I possibly alleviate my fears by turning my attention toward them?*

I had no trouble writing them down since I had so many, and the exercise itself prompted me to discover fears I didn't know I had. As with the resentments exercise, I had to acknowledge my part in the fears. In other words, what part of me was affected by the fear. It was an exercise in discovering that which I was trying to control. For example, my fear of taking risks was rooted in a fear of failure. Failure was threatening to my fragile ego and self-esteem, so I rarely took risks. Yet avoiding risks limited my potential for development and left me stagnant, frustrated, and resentful. I failed by default because I never tried, and in turn, I damaged my ego and self-esteem.

Instead of trying to avoid failure, I surrendered to it. I accepted all possible outcomes that would come from me trying something new. Surrender and acceptance relieved my fear of failure. Instead of running, I would experience the attempt, the risk, and any outcomes. Eliminating my fear of failure also relieved my anxiety and obsessions related to this particular fear. It was one of the most eye-opening experiences of my life.

Fear is a bully. It gains its strength from our attention to it. It loses strength when we recognize it for what it is: an overactive defense mechanism. The more we are able to acknowledge it as something dreamed up by our overly creative minds, the more it retreats, and the easier it is to move on.

While the fourth step exists in three parts, it was the section on fear where I made the greatest progress. Fear had anchored itself into my psyche since I was a child. It was the foundation of my anxiety and the most debilitating feature of my life. With a simple inventory, I found some level of peace from a thing that plagued me for as long as I can remember. I now had a powerful and effective tool to relieve my anxiety and remove irrational fear from my life. I could surrender control of the things I could not influence and find peace with it.

It was bravery through vulnerability, a vital step toward eliminating the fear completely. There is an enormous positive force behind vulnerability and honesty. While it initially makes us feel naked, exposed, and fearful, the growth and courage that come from it are immeasurable.

I realize that "letting go of fear" sounds overly simplistic and perhaps ambiguous. To be fair, it is more challenging than it sounds. For a person with anxiety, being afraid feels like we are a fly in a flytrap—the fear won't let us go. In reality, however, we are the flytrap, and we are holding on to the fear.

Letting go is less of an action to be taken and more of a behavior or habit to be formed through willingness and acceptance.

It is counterintuitive, but oftentimes, the reason we cannot let go of fear is because we aren't *willing* to let go of fear. Fear can protect us, but in many cases, it limits us. It can keep us from taking empowering steps beyond our comfort zone. For people like me, who are prone to excessive fear, it can be debilitating. When we finally realize that it is the fear itself causing us harm and not the thing the fear is supposedly protecting us from, we can become willing to let it go.

The final worksheet Jim gave me for my fourth step inventory had the word "HARMS" written along the top. I was to list out all of the people I had harmed and all the ways in which I had harmed them. It became clear to me why I had completed the resentments and fears lists first. Completing the resentments list opened my mind to my fault in each situation. The second list changed my relationship with fear. It was as if my spirit was being primed for the challenging tasks of acknowledging all of the situations where I had done people harm and finding the courage to face them. Had I done this exercise prior to completing the first two lists, my harms list would have been very short. Yet with willingness, an open mind, and a heart full of courage, the list was thorough.

It still wasn't easy to work through this list. It was painful to return to times when I had lied to my parents and watched my wife cry because of my actions. Of course, I returned to the accident that led me to this point. In my heart, I knew that this exercise was not a shameful one but an empowering one. I was cleaning up the wreckage of my past and forging a path to a new and wonderful life, much like the one that Jim was living. If I could just work through this, I could make things right with those I had wronged and then find peace in my own life. I could one day say the phrase I had longed to say and *mean*: "I've never had it so good!"

Completing the fourth step allowed me to begin coming to terms with who I really was. I was an alcoholic. I was a person who caused an accident while intoxicated. I was a person living with fear, anxiety, and shame. Most importantly, while those were facts about who I was, I didn't have to live with shame or suffering. I could get down to the business of changing that person to the person I wanted to become: a sober father and husband focused on continuous personal growth and healing. It was the step where things finally began to click for me, and the momentum I built carried on through the next steps. While steps five through twelve were not easy, they were not hard to tackle because I had the willingness to accomplish them, and I did so fearlessly— something I would have never been able to do on my own.

A community is key to recovery, and I was forging a solid community of sober mentors. In addition to AA and my sponsor, I began to take one-on-one therapy seriously, something I had not done in the past. I had been seeing a therapist for a few years, but I was far from honest or willing.

I would categorize my therapist as one of the most patient people in the world because I spent the majority of our time together lying and she knew it. She worked almost exclusively with addicts and knew our manipulative games all too well. I started with her because, during one of my brief periods of abstinence, my wife urged me (under the threat of divorce) to find a therapist. It was her belief that therapy would somehow get me to see the light and change my ways. While it worked for a time (during the period when I wanted to get the heat off), it ended up having the opposite effect over the long term.

It ended up providing me an alibi during my years of active alcoholism.

As long as I was attending therapy, I could effectively keep up the appearance that I was getting the help I needed while still drinking. The very fact that I was seeing a therapist gave me an avenue to play the victim—yet another avenue where I could divert responsibility from my myself for my behaviors.

How did it work out? Spoiler alert: not well.

I genuinely did want to work on my anxiety, but the therapy wasn't helping. My anxiety was getting worse. It wasn't the therapy that was failing me. I was failing myself because I continued to lie and manipulate my way back to a liquid solution. I was juggling all these lies with so many different people, and at some point, the house of cards would have to collapse.

When it finally did implode at the time of my DUI, the charade was over, and I became willing to let the therapy work.

Willingness didn't heal all wounds, but it did open the door to healing. I started being honest with my family, my therapist, and myself. Only through honest conversations did the tools I needed to overcome my anxiety finally start to take shape.

First, it was vulnerability that took the power away from anxiety. During an anxiety attack, I was conditioned to shut down and turn inward. I crumbled under the fear, and it became a downward spiral. The smaller I became, the larger the fear became. As I started opening up about my own story, the things I did, my shame, and my fears, the anxiety began to shrink; its power was less consuming. My bad thoughts couldn't thrive in isolation anymore. My family, friends, and community drowned out whatever my anxiety tried to convince me of. Vulnerability, community, and a willingness to heal became my weapons against anxiety. Honesty helped me heal.

It's counterintuitive to visualize something like vulnerability as a cure for anxiety. It seems as though becoming vulnerable would trigger our innermost fears. However, the monster of anxiety exists only in our heads. The nature of the anxiety is nearly always irrational. The monster is big, more than we can handle when we try to keep it in our heads. When we look to a supportive community and describe the monster that is terrorizing us in honest detail, the monster shrinks. We get out of our own heads and begin to observe the monster from outside ourselves, which allows us to see the monster as insignificant. The monster becomes the one who crumbles under the weight of honesty, community, and insignificance.

In my sickness, my brain told me negative, alarmist things to protect me in the moment, but in the long term, it led to greater harm. In the midst of an anxiety attack, my brain told me, "Keep this inside because people won't understand and they'll criticize you." The easy solution was to seek comfort in my addiction where I successfully numbed the pain in the present, but the long-term result was always more pain and suffering. Practicing vulnerability—opening up about my fears in a safe and compassionate space—was my new, sustainable solution.

It was opposite action, a practice of turning 180 degrees from what my brain was telling me and doing that. It's a careful art, because many times my brain may be telling me the truth. More often, my brain may be resigning to fear in an unhealthy way. It's at those times that opposite action is a necessary approach. For example, oftentimes I may be quiet and reserved. Sometimes that behavior is legitimate because I am an introvert and I need a break from people. On the other hand, if that quiet reservation is the result of an unhealthy motive such as self-pity or depression, I open up and tell people. I actively put myself in a state that contradicts the disempowering behavior. Doing this allowed my brain to develop new, healthy references for healing and growth.

All of these opposite actions taken against my disempowering thoughts served to thwart the monster of anxiety. They helped me understand that anxiety could be a superpower. Sure, anxiety, depression, and other mental disorders can be paralyzing and debilitating, but many of the psychological elements that make it so unbearable at their worst, are what make us powerful at our best. For every negative symptom of anxiety—the fear, obsessiveness, social awkwardness, and so on—there is an opposite positive symptom. A superpower.

For me, anxiety episodes had always been a chaotic roller-coaster of fight, flight, or freeze. Mostly it was flight and freeze as I retreated inwardly. I reinforced limiting beliefs and amplified my fears. As I began to practice the opposite action more and more, I also asked quality questions of myself. If anxiety reinforced limiting beliefs, I asked, "What if the opposite were true?" Episodes of anxiety were no longer hopeless. They were opportunities to be brave.

I once believed that people who performed courageous acts had no fear. What I came to understand as I learned more about my own superpowers was that courageous people do brave things in spite of the fear. Flipping the narrative and asking quality questions during periods of anxiety helped me discover new ways to shrink the anxiety monster. Specifically, when dealing with anxiety, I learned to ask myself the difficult question, "How can I perceive this negative condition or emotion in a positive way?"

Growing up, I was considered overly sensitive. Things tended to bother me more than they did other people, and I had a heightened sense of self-awareness. I kept tabs on how my actions and behaviors affected the world around me. I had always considered it a negative trait because it led me to become obsessive about what people thought of me. This hypersensitivity was, and still is, challenging in social situations.

Hypersensitivity manifests itself in social situations in interesting ways. In my case, I'm very conscious of how other people are feeling in the room. In other words, if the mood of the room is anxious, I will become anxious. If it is happy, I will feel happy. This used to trigger an obsessive reaction, where I constantly asked the people around me if they were all right. This often became quite annoying to the people around me. They found my incessant pestering annoying, not considerate.

Later I discovered that there is a name for this type of person. We are called empaths. It can be very exhausting, and it is a big reason why many people with social anxiety want to avoid large crowds, parties, and such. But with the right perspective, it can be an empowering attribute.

While getting sober, I asked myself, *How can I perceive this negative condition in a positive way?* While the sensitivity I feel can cause a disempowering obsession of what other people think of me, it can also mean that I have an enormous capacity to care for others, as long as I'm willing to be vulnerable and reach out. Cue the superhero music.

In AA, the desire to drink is often referred to as an obsession, and part of the spiritual awakening that we all strive for is to have the obsession lifted. Early in sobriety, I took this to mean that my obsessive nature would be removed. Later, I learned that it wasn't obsession itself that was removed, but the bond between my obsessive personality and alcohol. AA severed that bond and created a new bond between obsession and sobriety. My obsession with sobriety became a healthy obsession that didn't trigger negative effects, such as anxiety or depression. Instead, it was empowering.

For those of us with an obsessive nature, it is unreasonable to suggest that we can remove that nature completely, but we can realign our obsessive nature and create healthy bonds with sources of empowerment. It's not easy. In fact, the only way it was possible for me was when the incentive to form a healthy habit outweighed the benefits I thought I received from alcohol. It's difficult but not impossible.

Long before I understood any of this, I had already experienced linking my obsessive nature to something positive. When I played the cello in high school, I practiced for two to three hours a day without fail. It was a daily obsession that brought me joy and fulfillment. It filled me up rather than drained me. It was an obsessive focus that allowed me to grow and be my best, like my obsessive focus on sobriety later in life. Beyond sobriety, I applied obsessive focus, my superpower, in other positive areas as well.

An anxiety disorder doesn't get "cured." It doesn't go away, but we can learn to live with it. We can't reverse an obsessive personality, just as we can't expect someone to stop being sensitive, but these personality traits can be used for good.

In the first year of sobriety, I learned a lot about myself, how to manage my anxiety, and how to turn it into a superpower. I began to crave new and exciting experiences. I was no longer a cynic, but an optimist. In becoming an optimist, my luck began to change. Shifting my perspective toward what was possible kept me open to more positive experiences. The more positive experiences I witnessed, the better I perceived my luck to be.

With luck on my side, I felt a lust for new adventures. Adventure turned out to be yet another tool in my battle against anxiety. If there is a definitive cure for anxiety, I believe that adventure would be it. It stretches us beyond our limitations to show us our strength, resilience, and confidence.

Comfort Zone

IRONMAN ARIZONA, 2016. MILE 21.

For the first time in about an hour, I was finally able to stop pedaling. The sweet relief of a ten to fifteen mile stretch of false flat downhill was now before me, the same stretch that had just been a false flat uphill for the previous hour—the beginning of the out and back bike segment of Ironman Arizona.

A relatively flat bike course by Ironman standards, Ironman Arizona sends racers out of the town of Tempe out into the Sonoran Desert on a highway called the Beeline, and then they turn around in the middle of the desert and come back to Tempe. They do that loop three times.

The idea of a flat bike course is fantastic...in theory. I mean, what could possibly be better than a flat bike course? Well, lots of things, it turns out. In reality, a flat bike course can take a lot more out of a racer over the course of five hours. Without the gravity assist provided by downhill segments, one has to keep pressure on the pedals throughout the vast majority of the course. There is no opportunity to just let the wheels spin and get even the slightest bit of recovery.

Additionally, the lack of hills to break up a flat bike course doesn't offer racers much opportunity to get out of the aero position and stretch out their backs. I certainly could have got out of aero, but I would have also lost time to those who were willing to be uncomfortable longer than me.

Arizona had an additional mindfuck element to it. There was a gradual 1–3 percent grade all the way out into the desert. It was a demoralizing trip out of town, battling a slight uphill into the wind. The trip back to town, while slightly downhill and with the wind, didn't offer enough of a gravity assist to allow one to ease off the effort. The downhill was the opportunity to make up time lost on the uphill segment, not ease into comfort.

The six turnaround points were the only parts of the course where I stopped pedaling and got out of aero. I was at the first turnaround presently, and I fully embraced the four to five seconds of relief before getting back into the bars and grinding away.

As I felt my legs relax, the thought occurred to me that I could simply coast for a while. *What would it hurt?* I would still be making forward progress, and I would feel much more comfortable.

Ah, comfort...that manipulative bitch. The comfort zone would be so *comfortable*, but the comfort zone is an ever-changing target, always erring toward greater weakness, atrophy, and regression. If I let myself get comfortable now, I would leave time on the table. I would open the door to more comfort later. My "what-ifs" would remain "what-ifs."

I didn't get to my sixth Ironman starting line by being comfortable. I certainly wasn't going to let myself get comfortable until I crossed the finish line. Growth only happens outside of the comfort zone.

I put my head down, got back into the aero position, and resumed pedaling back toward town.

5

HOW TO CONVINCE YOUR WIFE THAT AN IRONMAN IS A GOOD IDEA

"You can learn a lot about life on the Big Island of Hawaii." These words came from the TV, which up until this point had only been background noise, spoken by a properly weathered voice—which I later discovered belonged to Al Trautwig. It was a couple months after I relapsed on the Big Island of Hawaii in 2006 that I first heard that iconic voice, and the word "Hawaii" elicited a Pavlovian response in me. When I heard it, my attention was immediately turned away from whatever I was doing at the time.

The screen displayed the Hawaiian coastline, erupting volcanoes, and waterfalls. I was immediately absorbed into the world unfolding before me. After my first trip to Hawaii back in 2000, I was obsessed with everything related to the state and tried to conceive of every possible way I could live there. Each time, I ended up talking myself out of it due to whatever fear and self-doubt decided to enter my mind at the time. When a TV show came on with iconic scenes of the Big Island, I was hooked. Al Trautwig's perfectly raspy narration combined with my fresh memories of our visit to the island just a couple months earlier only added to the experience.

Trautwig continued, "How it [life] can be rejuvenated to reveal what's deep inside..."

The words didn't have any special meaning to me at the time. It was the timbre and rhythm of the voice, along with the scenery, that held all the meaning for me. I wondered to myself what kind of travel documentary this could be.

"How boundaries are meant to be broken."

Then came a flawless segue from the enchanting scenery of the Big Island to a cannon blast, followed by a frenzy in the ocean. People were swimming on top of each other, fighting for breath and space. Then a group of people were cycling, drenched in sweat, and wearing grimaces on their faces. Feet pounded on the ground, while heat radiated from the pavement, all in dramatic, cinematic, slow motion.

"Those lessons come here in an event called the Ironman."

I'd heard about this Ironman thing before. I vaguely thought of it as some kind of 5K race or something. In that moment, I was about to learn exactly what it was. I discovered that I was watching a broadcast of the 2006 Ironman World Championship, the pinnacle of the sport of triathlon.

When I thought of the Ironman, I always pictured Speedo-clad Australians with perfect abs venturing out to do crazy things that Australians tend to do: ride a bike one hundred miles, sprint over a volcano, and wrestle a shark. You know, Wednesday for Australians.

"1,800 people, united by the challenge to prove, to inspire, and to finish a once thought to be unreachable distance."

Okay, here comes the shark wrestling part.

"Most of them are like you and me."

Bullshit, I thought. *Normal people can't do this.*

The narration then broke, and some of the athletes began listing their professions:

"Doctor, lawyer, teacher, marine, FBI agent, waitress..."

The list went on. These "normal" folks were about to swim 2.4 miles, ride a bike for 112 miles, and then run a full marathon, all in one day. There was nothing normal about that. In fact, there was everything crazy about that.

Then beyond the everyday people, I was introduced to the exceptional. Sister Madonna Buder, a seventy-six-year-old nun who was about to complete her twentieth Ironman. John Blais, who finished the Ironman a year earlier while battling ALS, was now spectating from a wheelchair. Dick and Rick Hoyt were a father and son team trying to finish for a second time. Rick Hoyt, afflicted with cerebral palsy, would be pulled and pushed through the race by his father, Dick. While they didn't make the cutoff in this version, they had completed the race back in 1989 in epic fashion.

There were countless stories like these, and I watched in awe, thinking to myself that this feat seemed impossible. Yet, here were people finishing the race with fucking smiles on their faces, even after seventeen hours.

I felt thoroughly inspired. These so-called "normal" people, some who were facing significant physical or psychological challenges, completed this seemingly impossible achievement. I thought for a moment how nice it would be to try to achieve something extraordinary like that. *How amazing would it be to stop drinking, get healthy, and finish an Ironman, inspiring my friends and family? Imagine what they would think of that. Imagine how I could transform my life. Imagine my joy.*

Then, I resigned myself to the reality of who I thought I was. To quit drinking, act bravely in spite of intense fear, exercise the discipline necessary to train for an event like this...It wasn't me.

I could never do something like that, I thought to myself.

I went out onto my patio and lit a cigarette, cracked another beer, and didn't think about Ironman again.

Until I did think about it again. Many years later, at the beginning of 2013, as I lay in bed recovering from a shoulder surgery, I let myself mull it over. It was a dumb injury, one which I deserved. I can't pinpoint the exact moment I was injured, but I know it was stupid. I know this because I had lived out most of my days up to that point neglecting physical activity that would improve my health. After all, I was young, and when we are young, we can eat oodles of pizza, drink gallons of beer, and inhale any number of carcinogens with zero consequences...or so I believed.

This was an odd conclusion to draw because I was also a nervous, hypochondriacal wreck who believed that everything bad was absolutely going to happen, definitely. A condition likely exacerbated by the consumption of said pizza, beer, and carcinogens.

Occasionally, I had fits of thinking, "I have to get my shit together," which led me to experiment with exercise. Because I was an ignorant alcoholic, I took exercise to the extreme. Instead of easing my way into it slowly, which would bring long-term success but require patience, I started where I wanted to end up, which was always aggressive and reckless. My thought was that I would not get the physique I wanted by going easy. No pain, no gain, as it is said, so I had to turn it up to eleven.

Naturally, I burned out rather quickly. Workouts became less energizing and more painful, and very quickly I would simply say "fuck it" and go back to channel surfing, only slightly more "swole" and much sorer.

This toxic mindset led me to the discovery of a successfully marketed "extreme" workout program in the mid-2000s. This program promised a shredded bod in ninety days. Ninety days? Yes! I loved exercise programs with an expiration date! What did I have to do to get the shredded bod? I had to spend every single one of those ninety days performing painful, anaerobic workouts with only the supervision and guidance of a two-dimensional celebrity workout instructor barking out orders from the television screen.

The goals of the program seemed arbitrary but tugged at the right macho chords for me at a time when the right mixture of low self-esteem, motivation, and desperation were present. "Learn how to do single-arm push-ups, jump squats, and weird crunch thingies! Why, you ask? Because *muscles*!"

Surprisingly, I actually completed the program. Not surprisingly, it came at a significant cost. With the absence of a healthy diet and the presence of a fairly persistent hangover, I didn't quite develop the shredded bod promised to me, and I quickly lost motivation and became burned out. Additionally, I felt the first indication of an unstable shoulder from the endless reps of pull-ups completed with terrible form. Like a trooper, I pressed on, only to make matters worse.

After I completed the program, my shoulder was too painful to continue with any exercise that involved lifting weights. Over the next few years, I used my bad shoulder as an excuse to forego the workouts and go to the Milk Duds. I descended deeper into self-pity. Painful, anaerobic exercise: 1; Adam: 0.

Fast forward to 2013. I was deeply immersed in repairing the wreckage of my past, while an orthopedic surgeon repaired the wreckage of my shoulder. With a year of sobriety, a year of psychological healing, and a new beginning of physical healing, I began to think about my physical well-being again. I began to ask myself, *What if?*

It's worth noting how important one year of sobriety is and what it meant to me. I had not had a full year of sobriety since I began my drinking career in my late teens. My previous experience with sobriety in 2006 ended at well under a year, and ever since that time, I had concluded that being sober for an entire year was an absolute impossibility.

Now I was nearly a full year sober, celebrating in anticlimactic fashion by lying in bed, recovering from surgery. Unglamorous as it was, it gave me plenty of time to reflect on the previous year, the lessons learned, and the opportunities that lay ahead.

In addition to my sober year, I was taking other steps toward a healthier life. A month prior, I put out my last cigarette. It wasn't hard to quit since I had learned some valuable lessons on how to quit obsessive behaviors. I had a complete willingness to do so and a set of tools to help me through it. In fact, I wanted to quit for many months, but my AA sponsor continued to overrule me with the "no major life changes for a year" speech. I respected his advice up until month eleven. With a surgery coming up in month twelve, where abstinence from nicotine would be forced on me, I decided to reduce my pain by quitting sooner rather than later. In retrospect, I am happy with that decision to go against my sponsor's advice.

My personal reflection on the previous year kept bringing me back to that important rule of sobriety: "Wait a year before you make any life changes." Now that I *had* a year, *what changes could I make?* This once seemingly impossible milestone was now accomplished, and it came without added anxiety, without an immediate desire to drink, and without pain. In fact, it was the exact opposite. The previous year, spent immersed in a culture of sobriety and positive action, led to an indescribable serenity, joy, and relief from anxiety. The questions then became: what seemingly impossible goal did I want to achieve next? What mountain did I want to climb? What unreachable distance did I want to run?

"Unreachable distance" triggered an emotion within me that brought me back to that Saturday afternoon in late 2006, when for one brief moment, I was inspired by normal people achieving an impossible dream. A desire was welling up inside of me. The images of athletes triumphantly crossing the Ironman World Championship finish line came pouring back into my mind. The harmony between these images and my present inspired state led to a dramatic epiphany that maybe, just maybe, I could become one of those finishers. It was an epiphany that was nearly severed by my next image. It was a vision of 2006 Adam dismissing this idea as absurd. As if traveling through time and space to greet me in 2013, cynical, drunk Adam chastised me for my absurd belief that I could compete in an Ironman. "You can never do that," 2006 Adam told me. "Just crack a beer and go back to feeling sorry for yourself."

"Bullshit," I said to 2006 Adam. "Yes, I fucking can."

The tools that I now had at my disposal, acquired through the experiences of the past year of sobriety, gave me the confidence and fortitude to tell 2006 Adam to go pound sand. Against that confidence, cowardly, afraid, drunken 2006 Adam whimpered away. I had found my life in sobriety. Now I was free to find my extra life. My extra life was going to begin with the Ironman Triathlon.

Not just any Ironman. I wanted to race *the* Ironman World Championship in Hawaii.

There are Ironman Triathlons, and then there is The Ironman World Championship on the Big Island of Hawaii. That is not to say that an Ironman by itself is an easy feat. Each of them offers a unique challenge, all covering 2.4 miles of swimming, 112 miles of cycling, and 26.2 miles of running. Yet I was transfixed on the *Hawaii* Ironman, and I was dead set on getting into that race.

It didn't take me long to learn that getting a slot in the Hawaii Ironman would be...a challenge, to put it mildly. There were a few ways in which I could get into the race. The first was by qualification. Each race had a predetermined number of qualifying spots, usually between thirty and seventy-five total, handed out to the top finishers of each age group. With over two thousand participants in each race, the number of qualifiers per race was, at best, 4 percent of the total participants. To add to this difficulty, as a male in my early thirties, I was going to be in one of the most competitive age groups, the thirty to thirty-four age group. The number of qualifiers between the ages of thirty to forty could shrink to as low as 1 percent of total participants, or three out of three hundred athletes. Many people who qualify between the ages of thirty to fifty are either (a) former professionals at one of the three disciplines (swimming, biking, or running), (b) fitness coaches, (c) lifelong athletes, or (d) mutants. I was none of these things. It was extremely rare for a dark horse with zero experience in any of the three disciplines, and a gut full of cheeseburgers, to finish on the podium of an Ironman Triathlon, which is what it would take to secure a world championship slot.

To put it into perspective, in many Ironman races (depending on many different variables, such as weather, course terrain, etc.), a podium mostly includes athletes finishing anywhere between eight and a half hours on the low end to ten hours on the high end. This would typically mean having to swim 2.4 miles in about an hour, bike 112 miles in less than five hours, and run a full marathon in under three and a half hours. For those who may not be familiar with what those times mean relative to the distances of each discipline, I'll summarize by saying it's really freaking fast.

I had zero experience in triathlons. I had told nobody about my new desire and anticipated that it would draw a hell of a laugh from friends and family, which I would fully deserve given my present state. I had no business believing I could do an Ironman Triathlon, but the picture I painted in my mind was very real. I imagined running down the finisher's chute on Ali'i Drive with a smile on my face and giving a slow-motion fist pump at the finish line.

If I'm being honest, I even visualized myself as one of the athletes featured on the television broadcast I had once seen. Qualifying for Ironman Hawaii would be hard enough; it was a stretch to think I would be one of the athletes filmed for the broadcast. Given how hard it is to even qualify for Kona, only a select few are actually featured on the show—but a boy could dream, regardless of how ridiculous the dream is. I not only wanted to demonstrate to myself that I could achieve anything I put my mind to, but I wanted to demonstrate to the world that there was a life beyond the bottle and joy beyond anxiety. I had never even ridden a road bike, barely swam the length of a pool without gasping for air, and always got winded halfway up a flight of stairs, but I saw myself crossing the Ironman finish line more clearly than I had ever seen anything else in my life. A dream was born.

For the time being, however, I kept this dream close to the vest.

The big secrecy stemmed back to an experience my wife, Marie, and I had shortly after we moved into our first apartment after college. We decided it would be fun to buy mountain bikes as a way to acquaint ourselves with our new environment. We went out and bought a couple of low-end mountain bikes and decided to take them out for a test ride on our local trails.

Now, these were not single-track, double black diamond advanced trails. These were about as beginner as they could get. Granted, Marie and I certainly did fit the description of beginner, opting for the cheapo mass-produced mountain bikes rather than a slick specialty bike with more zeros on the price tag. Shortly into our ride, we were stopped by a man who was clearly many tens of thousands of dollars farther into the sport than we were. He first warned us of a swarm of bees up ahead on the trail, but then he questioned our experience level. As he dug in, he began critiquing our bikes, our matching helmets, and our capabilities. He seemed to have cued into our vulnerabilities as novice riders and dug the knife in deep. He laughed at our naïveté under the guise of being helpful. We turned around humiliated and went home. Our bikes remained in storage for nearly a decade. I went away from that experience believing that the endurance world was exclusive and closed off.

Thanks to this negative interaction, I believed that telling anyone about my new dream would result in a condescending, "Well, good for you!" at best, and more likely, "That's the dumbest idea I've ever heard," followed by unceasing laughter. I had to keep this a secret, if at the very least to keep the dream alive.

There was one exception. Marie had stuck with me through everything. Surely I could reveal my new and crazy dream to her. She was safe. If she shut it down immediately, at least it would be honest and loving, and I would have my out. I needed someone to grab my legs and pull me back down to Earth so that I didn't risk another humiliating failure that was doomed from the start.

There was also the small chance that she would approve, in which case, I would have to follow through and commit myself to actually learn how to swim, bike, and run. I would have to complete the damn thing or kill myself trying.

Shit.

I considered the many ways in which I could bring the subject of Ironman up.

"Hi, honey. Do you need anything at the store? Toilet paper? Apples? An Ironman Triathlon?"

Or I could take a more subtle approach and leave a YouTube video of an Ironman race up on her computer screen so that when she opened it, I could casually walk by and say, "What is this that you're watching? Ironman Triathlon, hmm? Wouldn't it be a hoot if I signed up for one of those?"

Nah, I had to just open up the can and lay the contents out on the table. *If it's meant to be, it's meant to be*, I thought.

As the scenarios surrounding the conversation rolled around in my head, I pictured a lot of outcomes. One scenario in particular went something like this:

Me: "So, I want to do an Ironman."

Marie: "You what?"

Me: "Let me start over..."

Marie: "Good idea."

Me: "I once saw the Ironman Triathlon on TV, and I want to do it."

Marie: "You want to try something just because you saw it on TV? Isn't that something we try to steer our kids away from?"

Me: "Okay, I see your point. Take three..."

I couldn't think of a good way to bring up the subject that didn't make me sound crazy. I took a deep breath and thought a little harder. *Why did I really want to pursue this? Why not just be honest and tell my wife what prompted me to become so focused and passionate about this goal that had never even been on my radar until now?*

When I finally mustered the courage to speak to her about my new dream, I learned I severely underestimated the enthusiasm with which my wife wants to support me.

"I've been working on my sobriety for the past year," I told her. "During that time, I've been able to overcome my obsession with alcohol and develop ways to manage anxiety and depression. These are things I never would have thought possible. I feel like I can do more."

I went on to tell her the story about the time I watched the Ironman Triathlon on TV. I told her about the distances involved, how I originally thought those people were crazy, and how I believed that I could never do something like that until I achieved something else that I thought was impossible: sobriety.

"So, you want to compete in an Ironman Triathlon?" she asked.

"Yes," I responded. "It came to me like an epiphany that I can do this. I've always been afraid, anxious, and worried about everything. It's because of this that I've never tried anything new, traveled the world, or taken risks. It's one of the reasons that I kept going back to drinking. I was afraid and resentful of myself for never trying things or participating in life. I realize now, since I've removed these negative aspects from my life, that I can do the things I once thought were impossible. It's not just about competing in an Ironman; it's about recognizing a fear I once had and overcoming it. Because I *can*."

"Are you done?" she asked.

"Um, yeah."

"Good. I think it's an awesome idea!"

I couldn't believe she was so quick to support the idea. I had four and a half more pages of speech to get through.

Her look then turned inquisitive. "How do you get started?"

I thought for a moment. "That is a good question..."

Her eyes then lit up. "When do we get to go to Hawaii?"

Sugar Water

IRONMAN BOULDER, 2015. MILE 92.

As my watch buzzed for what seemed like the zillionth time during this race, my face grimaced and turned green. Once again, the buzzing was the signal to take a swig from my lemon-lime concentrated sugar water concoction I called "race nutrition." In every other race up to this point, the blend had served me well, but this time was different.

My eleven-year-old self would have jumped at the opportunity to chug super concentrated lemonade. Hell, my thirty-year-old self would have jumped at the opportunity. Ninety miles into this Ironman, it was the last thing I wanted.

My stomach had been upset ever since I got out of the Boulder Reservoir after completing the swim portion of the race. I'm not sure if it was leftover nerves from before the race, the fact that I inadvertently drank or inhaled about a third of the water within the reservoir during my swim lap around it, the altitude, or some combination of the three, but my gut was mad at me, and it would not shut up about it.

I begrudgingly grabbed my bottle from the downtube of my bike and took a big sip, followed by a large gulp of water. I could feel that my stomach was about to retaliate so I slowed to a stop on the side of the road and allowed myself to recover a bit. I couldn't afford to vomit up the nutrition I had taken in. Going into a marathon with a major calorie deficit was a big no-no.

I gazed up at the road ahead. It was a steep incline going far into the distance, beyond where the eye could see. It was a series of hills affectionately referred to as "The Three Bitches." I don't know exactly how that name was established, but by just looking at it, it wasn't difficult to determine how it got its name.

The brief pause on the side of the road gave my stomach a chance to settle. Unfortunately, just because I had been successful in keeping the drink down didn't mean that it was providing me the energy I needed. It was simply sloshing around in my belly like a shitty water jug in my abdomen. It was a sure sign that my digestive system had told me to go fuck myself and shut down completely.

I weighed my options. I could throw everything up and start from scratch with an empty stomach, but then, of course, I would have the calorie deficit issue. I could suck it up and power through, but that would probably lead to a massive meltdown on the run.

One thing was certain at that moment: I fucking hated sugar water and wanted nothing to do with it. This opinion was a massive departure from my feeling hours ago when I would have given my left testicle (and probably my right one also after enough negotiation) for a donut. My diet had been so meticulous and so disciplined that I avoided added sugar altogether up to race day. Now it was like the devil was inviting me to have my fill, and thanks to the nasty lake water, I was begging for a reprieve.

It was an ironic twist of fate. After all this effort over time to become healthy, to avoid sugar, and to prepare myself for these extreme endurance challenges, I ended up binge drinking straight refined sugar in order to provide instant energy during physical exertion, and it was making me sick to boot.

I have prepared for this. I will not be taken down now.

I was reminded at that moment of how good my clean diet made me feel. How much easier it was to exercise after eating nutrient-rich, fresh foods instead of processed junk. How much more energy I had than before. How I felt light instead of heavy. How that clean diet gave me the foundation to train as well as I could, which got me to this point in an Ironman freaking Triathlon. I may have felt sick as a dog, but I got this far because of new healthy habits. If I hadn't adopted those healthy habits, I would have never made it to the start line.

I pressed on, inspired by my renewed belief that I could make it to the finish line because of the person I had become, not the person I was.

6

RIP CHEESEBURGERS

had to be smart about this. I mean, seriously. The very reason
I was lying in bed, recovering from surgery in the first place,
was because I was *not* smart about health and fitness. I had
resolved to do an Ironman, a resolution I made quite literally
at the peak of unhealthiness. I couldn't let myself sabotage my
new goal. I knew a little research would be prudent so as not
to risk my heart exploding out of my chest whilst jogging at a
pace that was way above my capabilities just because I thought
it was the pace I needed to run.

Fortunately, fate dealt me a hand (or rather an injured shoulder) that forced me to be patient and considerate about training
for an Ironman, but boy, was it hard to stifle the urge to just get
out and start training.

Now that my heart was set on doing an Ironman and I had
the support of my wife, the obsession to begin training was

welling up inside of me. Doctor's orders, however, were that I avoid swimming, biking, and running for at least six weeks, which up until about three days earlier, was no problem. Can't swim, bike, or run? Done, done, and done! Now hand me another donut!

But now I was a triathlete in training. *How could I ever expect to become Ironman-ready if I wasn't able to actually do the three disciplines? What if all this motivation just melted away within the next six weeks of medically imposed laziness?* Typical alcoholic thinking. We have no desire to do something until we physically can't do it, and then it becomes our life's obsession. Very funny, universe.

In truth, though I believed it to be a huge inconvenience at the time, it was a blessing in disguise. It prevented me from making the same mistake I had made so many times before: acting on my initial motivation with aggressive exercise to the point of destroying my body, burning out, giving up, and then descending back into unhealthy habits. This time I had the capacity, flexibility, and time to develop a plan of action.

What was I to do in these six weeks of sloth? I knew what I couldn't do. What I could do was learn. Learning was one thing I was really good at when I was on an obsessive streak. In fits of obsessiveness, I absorbed information like a sponge, and as a result, it kept me motivated. With all my free time, that's what I did. I started researching triathlon training. But more than triathlon training, I wanted to learn how to be as healthy and fit as possible. I didn't just want to finish a triathlon; I wanted to rise above chronic unhealthiness and become sustainably healthy and a peak performer. For the first time in my life, free from the grips of alcoholism and addiction, I was in a position where there was nothing preventing me from developing a world-class healthy lifestyle. *That* was my primary goal. The test would be Ironman.

Additionally, I could stop eating like a scumbag immediately. Up to that point, I had been a notoriously terrible eater. I always started my day off strong with a fruit smoothie. Back in college, I read a book that said that starting your day off with fruit was a good way to combat anxiety. It was a compelling enough message for me to implement it and imprint it as a habit for many years. Oddly, it didn't seem to have the positive effect the book promised, but I was convinced that if I broke the habit, my anxiety would get even worse. Anxiety is exhausting.

Regardless, it didn't really matter how I started my day, because after that first smoothie, it was game on for all kinds of junk food. From fast food to obsessive snacking on candy and soda, my blood was probably about 70–80 percent high fructose corn syrup. With a new healthy outlook, it was time to say goodbye to cheeseburgers.

And other things.

I didn't just want to single out cheeseburgers. Cheeseburgers get a bad rap. Let's face it: they're delicious and not the worst offender. It is possible to find a healthy cheeseburger, but not from the sources from which I was getting them. Still, they were just one of many, many, many things that I put in my mouth, and subsequently swallowed, which would contribute to the constriction of my arteries, expansion of my gut, and the shortening of my life.

It was time to get to work, but the difficult question I had to answer was where to start. Typing "healthy diet" into a search engine opens up a firehose of search results, ranging from useless clickbait to gimmicky, short-term solutions. Furthermore, each website sent me down a rabbit hole of conflicting information.

"Count calories!"

"Don't count calories. Focus on macros!"

"Carbohydrates are the devil!"

"Consume more coconut oil!"

"Don't consume coconut oil!"

It was enough to make my head spin. No wonder people fail at dieting. All they find are short-term solutions that force them to second-guess every food-related decision. Who could I trust?

It dawned on me that perhaps the best approach was to simplify. Before I went too far with any strategy, I decided to grab the low-hanging fruit, both figuratively and literally.

Inherently, I think everyone knows the difference between good food and bad food. I knew that I needed to eat more vegetables and fruits and less candy bars. That became step one. I just started eating the obviously healthy stuff and avoided the obviously unhealthy stuff. "Reduce the complexity and simplify" became my new mantra. If it wasn't simple, it wasn't sustainable, and I needed sustainability to be successful.

While the approach seemed simple—eat more obviously healthy natural foods and less processed junk food—it would be far from easy. If changing a habit was as simple as just stopping the bad thing and doing the good thing, there would be far fewer problems in the world today. Sadly, my bond with junk food was equally as strong as my bond with alcohol. At least now I had a reference point for breaking a bond with alcohol. Could I do the same with junk food?

The idea of adding healthy foods to my diet wasn't much of a problem. I could supplement my meals with salads, fruits, nuts, and all sorts of other foliage without much resistance or gagging. It was the removal of the added sugar (sugar that doesn't naturally occur within the food itself) and other processed foods with complex ingredients that became more difficult.

The obviously unhealthy stuff was hard enough to eliminate. Over a long period of time, I had created strong emotional attachments and obsessive habits around fast food, potato chips, candy, ice cream, cookies, and more. I was already struggling just to imagine life without these comfort foods. The not-so-obvious unhealthy foods only made it more difficult.

While strolling the aisles at the grocery store, I began a practice that I had never done before. I began looking at the nutrition label of food items.

Up to that point, I usually checked the front of the box or jar first. If a pleasant picture of a cartoon cheese puff or similarly stunning anthropomorphic representation of a food item appealed to me, I moved on to step two: look at the price tag. If the price was attractive enough, followed by enough exclamation points, and outlined by a comic book explosion icon, I was sold.

What can I say? I like cartoons.

Now that I was investigating food items further, I was surprised and demoralized to discover that many of these items contained either added sugar, ingredients I didn't recognize, or both. Even some of the non-cartoonish foods I thought were healthy contained high amounts of sugar or strange ingredients. Items like healthy cereals, pasta sauces, and canned vegetables...I mean, *canned vegetables*!

It all made me realize that throughout the course of my life, I consumed dangerous amounts of sugar that I didn't know about, on top of the dangerous amounts of sugar that I *did* know about.

The seemingly simple action of removing unhealthy processed foods from my diet proved to be very difficult from an emotional standpoint. Much like alcohol prior to my recovery, junk food and poor dietary habits were anchored within my psyche and served as a coping mechanism, a comfort, and a source of immediate gratification. Much of the food that I discovered to be unhealthy elicited an overpowering sense of loss when I thought of eliminating them.

With alcohol, when I was drinking, if I did not have alcohol nearby, I missed it terribly. The same was true for my favorite junk foods. I felt a sense of loss when they weren't around. The bond between my obsession and junk food was strong and, like alcohol, needed to be broken. But as was true about my bond with alcohol, it couldn't be broken by willpower alone.

Breaking the emotional attachment to food required a change in psychology, not just restriction or abstinence. I couldn't just go on a diet like so many people with uncompelling goals. I needed sustainability. I wanted this lifestyle to *last*. I wanted to qualify for the Ironman World Championship. That required a level of discipline above and beyond an empty resolution to just eat healthier.

Every piece of food that entered my mouth needed to serve a purpose. It had to serve the goal of who I wanted to become. I had to let go of my emotional relationship with food in order to develop a *functional* relationship with food. Before I could develop a functional relationship with food, I first had to understand my emotional relationship so that I could effectively break the bond. *What was it that drove me to obsessively and compulsively desire and eat junk food?*

I fixated so intensely on the "what" of my diet—the unhealthy versus the healthy foods—I had never really considered the "why."

When I dug deep enough into the reasons why I ate the way that I did, I realized that I simply wanted what everyone wants: to be happy and fulfilled. Yet, I didn't have a compelling vision of what my long-term happiness looked like. It was just a weak notion in my mind that someday I would be happy. Without that compelling vision for long-term happiness and fulfillment, the only option was to find a short-term solution. Food was an easy option because it provided immediate gratification. If I was feeling down, food was there to comfort me. If I was anxious, food was there. Bored? Food! Lonely? Food! The strong emotional attachment was formed.

Now I had a dream. I was going to be an Ironman and qualify for the world championship. It was a belief so strong that it became my compelling purpose to sever the emotional bond to food and form a strong functional bond. I also had sobriety, a point of reference so powerful it led me to believe I had the ability and discipline to achieve anything I set my mind to. My mind was now set on eating a clean, functional diet.

Our pantry was emptied of the processed foods, juices, and sodas and filled with produce, nuts, high-quality meats, and olive oil. No calorie counting, no complex gimmicky diets, just simple, clean foods eaten to the point of satisfaction.

After the initial period of detox from junk food, which was admittedly painful, I experienced a dramatic improvement in my mood, energy, and physical state. The headaches from sugar withdrawal faded. The sugar cravings were satisfied by eating an apple (or sometimes two or three). I thought that I would not see any significant physical transformation until I started increasing physical activity. I was wrong. The greatest improvement to my physical and mental condition came as a result of changes to my diet, even though I was in a sedentary state, still recovering from my shoulder surgery.

Over time, I discovered that simple foods were often not only delicious, but life transforming. I began to actually taste the rich flavors of fruits and vegetables I was eating, and I started to enjoy preparing tasty, healthy meals. There was also a sense of satisfaction that came with eating a healthy meal, which was a change from the persistent obsession of eating beyond being full. Satisfaction became the new "full," and it meant an end to caring about the number of calories on a plate.

Once I started a healthy diet rich in fruits and vegetables and free from copious amounts of refined sugar, I no longer had to count calories. I ate until I was satisfied, and that was enough. I better regulated my food intake thanks to proper biofeedback, clear of any toxic amount of refined sugar.

Think about it. How often do we hear about someone lacking control over the amount of kale or celery they could consume?

In the same spirit of discovery in which I found a life without alcohol to be freeing, I found a life without excess sugar freed me from the bonds of fatigue and relieved anxiety and depression. The discipline of healthy eating brought me freedom. As badass Navy SEAL Jocko Willink said, "Discipline equals freedom."

Even though I wasn't yet exercising, within the first month alone of the change in diet habits, I lost fifteen pounds. The initial focus on why I wanted to end my emotional relationship with food and develop a functional relationship with food—followed by enacting simple, clean, sustainable nutritional habits—led to my success. Simplifying my diet gave me the flexibility and capacity to focus on improving my mindset toward food and ultimately increased my chances of success.

It was serendipitous that I was able to get my diet under control while recovering from a surgery that didn't allow me to do any exercise. It forced me into a proper state of humility where

I was open to learning everything I could. I learned how to manage my diet, and at the same time, I learned what I had to do to begin training for the Ironman. Instead of jumping right into aggressive, painful, and often injurious training, I was forced into patience, which was a huge blessing in disguise.

Serendipity became a theme for me. As I started down a healthier, more optimistic path, my luck changed. I met with the right people and discovered new secrets to sustainable health and fitness. In the coming years, my life would continue to transform for the better.

Walking

IRONMAN BOULDER, 2015. MILE 125.

"Are you okay?" asked Ironman champion Tim Don.

I didn't know it was Tim Don at the time, mostly because I didn't know who Tim Don was. I learned about him well after this race as I watched Mr. Don on television set a world record in a Brazilian Ironman. As I discovered it, I immediately exclaimed, "Dude! That's the guy who asked me if I was okay during Ironman Boulder!" But at this particular moment, I had no idea who he was.

"Yeah, I'm fine," I replied.

I was not fine. I had about fifteen more miles to "run" in this race, which was quickly becoming a test of survival. I couldn't do any better than a walk. I stopped by an aid station to grab some Gatorade and water, and as I sipped on each, I swayed from side to side.

Ironman Boulder was a unique course because of the number of professional triathletes in attendance. Most of these pros were among the spectators, not the competitors. Since Boulder, Colorado, is home to many pro athletes, they come out to cheer on the age groupers—the non-pros who had paid for the right to participate in this torture. I was not putting on a great show for them...or maybe I was. It really depends on the perspective.

"Well, keep on going! You're doing great!" Tim Don lied as I stumbled on.

I must have looked like death at this moment. I was physically beat because I had just put myself through over a hundred miles of hell, and I was mentally dejected as I realized the many miles I still had to cover to make it to the finish line.

Quitting never entered my mind, though. Even if I had to crawl to the finish line, I was going to make it. Even if it would be my worst finish yet, I was going to press on. There were people in this race who were going to battle to make the midnight cutoff, and they would be ecstatic to do so. There were people overcoming significant challenges, and they were the ones who inspired me. That was my reason for pressing on, and I wasn't going to let a tough day beat me. I was going to finish, and I was going to do so with a smile on my face.

I began to hazard a jog, just to see if I could maintain it. As I did, I heard a dog barking. It sounded like Charlie.

Poor Charlie.

Charlie was our yellow Labrador Retriever, the sweetest dog in the world, who we had just put down prior to our trip to Boulder. I began to cry as I thought about him. I felt like Charlie was barking at me now, telling me to keep moving forward, willing me on, and saying that everything was okay and that he forgave me for having to end his life.

I tend to get emotional during the second half of an Ironman marathon.

It did give me a second wind, and I continued a steady, albeit slow, jog. It was a jog that would be frequently broken up by long periods of walking, but that certainly wasn't something that was new to me. I was familiar with walking.

7

THE
FOUNDATION

was getting frustrated. After years of desiring nothing more than to take the path of least resistance, which often involved me on the couch eating nachos, I finally *wanted* to work out. I wanted desperately to swim, bike, and run, but I could do none of these things. At the command of my doctor, I was only allowed to walk.

Walk I did. A lot. I was determined to become the best walker in the world. It was actually very enjoyable and foreshadowed the inevitable path I would come to follow in my Ironman training. It was a path of humility and acceptance, and it was an important hurdle to overcome. It was my meditation, and it made me feel refreshed, energized, and alive.

The energy I gained gave me loads of positive side effects. It got my obsessive juices flowing, and I was able to channel those obsessive juices into researching triathlon training. After all, if I were going to legitimately do this Ironman thing, and not die of stupidity, I needed to figure out how to go about it.

The hardest part about anything is knowing where to start. I had no clue how to even look for the right type of information. I read tons of blogs from athletes, race reports, and the like, all with the goal of getting some hint of how I should begin, but all of these folks were already rock star triathletes. I needed a beginning. I started digging deeper, learning the stories of successful Ironman athletes to whom I could relate, and trying to dissect how those people did it. I started with YouTube, watching videos of old Ironman World Championships to find those unicorn stories. I worked my way backward from the race the previous year (2012) and just absorbed the stories, professional triathletes and amateurs (also known as "age groupers") alike, trying to find some glimmer that these athletes were once human, and not just genetic wonders. I hoped to model their growth instead of killing myself to achieve some unrealistic goal. I kept searching until I stumbled upon a defining event in the history of Ironman: The Iron War.

The Iron War between Dave Scott and Mark Allen in the 1989 Ironman World Championship is arguably the most notable event in triathlon history. For many years, Mark Allen was chasing an elusive victory at the iconic race, yet he repeatedly fell apart and lost. Meanwhile, Dave Scott dominated, winning six world championships throughout the eighties.

Until 1989.

Allen made some changes to his training the year leading up to the Hawaii Ironman in 1989, and he was ready to face Scott once again. This time, Allen did not fade. For the entire race, Allen stayed with Scott as they battled for the lead. It's one thing to be neck-and-neck in a hundred-yard sprint, but it's an entirely different and infinitely more awkward thing to be racing shoulder to shoulder for eight hours, not saying a word to one another. The tension could be cut with a knife, and the result was an exciting climax late in the race.

Allen matched Scott step for step on the run until something magical happened with less than five kilometers left to go. Allen broke away, and Scott could not catch him. Allen won. He finally defeated his Goliath.

Mark Allen went on to win five more Ironman World Championships before hanging up his Oakleys in the mid-nineties.

What was it that so dramatically changed about Allen's training that took him from falling apart to breaking an Ironman record and becoming a repeat champion five more times? Did Allen discover some secret formula that allowed him to turn his fitness around? If so, was this a formula that a mere mortal like myself could employ?

It turns out the secret was absurdly simple. He slowed down.

Under the guidance of coach Phil Maffetone, Allen learned the art of heart rate training for aerobic endurance. Maffetone's approach, appropriately called the "Maffetone Method," involved doing the majority of training under a maximum aerobic heart rate, under which the greatest endurance adaptations can be made. According to Maffetone, the maximum aerobic heart rate is found simply by subtracting the athlete's age from 180—plus or minus a few points, depending on current fitness—and voila! That's the secret formula (*The Big Book of Endurance Training*, 2010).

That's it? I thought. *Really?*

Yes, really. It turns out, most of us are so convinced that if we don't "feel" the pain of our workouts, we miss out on some of the best fitness gains we could possibly achieve. We are brainwashed by the idea of "no pain, no gain," so we burn out, get injured, and lose motivation. Such was the story of my failed fitness career up to that point.

The purpose behind the Maffetone Method is to develop a strong fat-burning engine by employing aerobic effort. Did that mean that I dressed up in my finest eighties leotard and danced to Belinda Carlisle's "Mad About You"? Not quite. Aerobic workouts in this sense referred to an energy system within the body, not an outdated exercise fad.

During exercise, people are always burning some combination of glycogen (the "fast burning" energy of which there are limited stores in our bodies) and fat (the "slow burning" energy of which we have plentiful stores). In many cases, when a person is exercising, an anaerobic response is triggered when effort increases to a significant degree, at which time the body starts burning a higher percentage of glycogen than fat. This is accompanied by increased respiration and heart rate. Because human beings have a finite supply of glycogen stores within their bodies (about two thousand calories), we can't maintain this effort for extended periods of time.

As a primarily sedentary individual who consumed massive amounts of sugar and rarely exercised, my body was conditioned to immediately engage the anaerobic system. My body believed that the only reason I would be running is if someone chased me, so it responded as such. The result was a lot of huffing and puffing and massive burnout.

When training *aerobically*, one is using oxygen as the primary source of energy and using a higher percentage of fat for fuel. This, in turn, increases our capacity to burn fat as we gradually develop endurance. Fat is the most efficient fuel we have. It is the energy store we use for sustained effort over very long periods, meaning many hours or days. A person with a well-conditioned aerobic system could run for hours, completing a marathon, triathlon, or even an Ironman.

Theoretically, by training at a very slow pace under the maximum aerobic heart rate that the Maffetone Method prescribed, I could condition my body to burn fat as a primary source of fuel. Over time, as my fitness developed, I would get faster and stronger under that same heart rate, which would allow me to cover a greater distance without tapping into critical glycogen stores. Thus, I could avoid the dreaded "bonk" (also known as "hitting the wall").

Mark Allen transformed his racing career through this simple change in strategy, and he became the world's best endurance athlete. I wondered what it could do for me.

When I learned about Allen's story, it resonated with me deeply. I remembered the initial motivation I would have to go out and exercise, and then I remembered the burnout I would feel after just a few days of working out. I recalled the pain, the injury, and the demoralizing fatigue that would accompany my athletic pursuits. It got to the point where I believed that exercise just wasn't good for me. I recollected that nothing seemed to help me feel better, and that the claims of exercise calming anxiety and depression were all a load of bullshit.

Maybe I just need to slow down, I thought.

I concluded that it was worth testing out this philosophy since any immediate future recovery protocol related to my shoulder would require easy exercise anyway. I thought I might as well buy a heart rate monitor to start applying the Maffetone Method once I got the go-ahead from the doctor.

I forked over the forty dollars to purchase a heart rate monitor from Amazon and waited. In the meantime, I was about to start physical therapy, which meant I could get myself out of this damn sling and start strengthening my arm.

Physical therapy meant something entirely new. Progress. For weeks, I had been sitting in limbo, just researching triathlons obsessively and waiting to be well enough to start doing something besides walking. While the exercises were simple, such as lifting a broomstick into the air and then putting it down again, it was *something*, and it was progress.

It's funny because nowadays when people say to me that they could never train for an Ironman because they don't know how to swim, bike, or run, or whatever excuse du jour, I always remember my first step of the Ironman journey began by lifting a broomstick. I didn't know how to swim, bike, or run properly, and I sure as hell didn't know how to put them together. All I was *allowed* to do was lift a broomstick and walk. But doing just those things was progress. Regardless of one's limitations or obstacles in the way of a goal, every journey starts with the same thing: action. No matter how big or small, an action toward a goal spurs momentum and progress.

I had been through physical therapy in the past. I suffered a neck injury that resulted in a ruptured cervical disk. This injury required a fusion of my C6–C7 vertebrae, another result of being overly ambitious when it came to physical activity. That first experience with physical therapy led me to believe that it was a necessary evil required by insurance companies so that they could avoid the expense of a surgery. The facility then seemed like a factory. There were dozens of people getting worked on by machines, and only two or three therapists walked around to check on the clients. I was hooked up to a traction machine and left to stare at the ceiling. It was a painful experience, both physically and mentally.

This time, however, I was assigned to a more unassuming therapist. I walked into the office, and a man greeted me at the front. He introduced himself as Cal. He immediately took me to the back room and began working on my shoulder. He talked to me about my injury. He described in detail the muscles that were involved and *why* we were strengthening them. It was so simple for him to explain to me why an exercise was needed and how it was being done so that I could understand my healing. There were no machines, only personal one-on-one attention.

In a word, Cal cared.

I was impressed with the photos and sports memorabilia adorning the walls. He had autographed pictures of figure skaters, hockey players, and cyclists. Right below one of the pictures, a road bike leaned up against the wall. This piqued my interest.

"So, you're a cyclist?" I asked.

"Yes, I do quite a bit of riding," he replied. "Do you ride?"

The question threw me for a loop. I didn't ride, of course, but after a few weeks of obsessively watching Ironman videos, learning about bikes, and reading up on all of the training resources available (which was a lot), I could only muster a somewhat awkward answer. "I *really* want to, but I never have."

I was afraid to talk about my ambitions with this random stranger, but this was probably exactly the person I needed to talk to about them. I started asking questions again.

"What kind of cycling do you do?" I asked.

He responded that he did some group rides in the area, some advanced rides with semi-pro athletes. But what caught my attention was the fact that he had participated in triathlons in the past.

"Have you ever heard of Wildflower?" he asked, to which I responded I hadn't. "It's a 70.3 in central California, with tons of climbing, but it's a lot of fun."

"A 70.3?"

"Yes," he replied. "It's a half-iron distance triathlon. A 1.2-mile swim, 56-mile bike, and a 13.1-mile run."

He went on to describe how challenging the event was. All the climbing on the bike, the hills on the run, and the heat. People camped out before the race and made a party out of it. It had a bit of a cult following. I was enthralled.

The conversation ended for the day, and I left with my new broomstick exercises. I was still reluctant to tell anyone of my desire to do an Ironman, especially a physical therapist who had literally been a triathlete. Honestly, my ego was getting the best of me.

It was easy to recognize my hesitancy as alcoholic thinking. Surely, Cal would not hear my desire to compete in an Ironman Triathlon and immediately laugh me out of his office, but my brain still had that fear, rooted within my ego, and it inhibited me from being vulnerable. Though I no longer had a desire to drink, the alcoholic thinking could still creep in. At least I had the understanding and tools to recognize it, even if I didn't immediately address it. As it is often said in the rooms of recovery, the program is about progress, not perfection.

Over time, as I warmed up to Cal, I broached the subject a little bit more. I told him that I read up on the Wildflower, and it looked awesome. I told him what I knew about Mark Allen and Phil Maffetone. Finally, after a few sessions, I told him that I was thinking about signing up for an Ironman. Cal was officially the second person I told.

"That's awesome," he said. "I have resources that might help you. And when you do buy a bike, let me know because I can give you a bike fit."

A bike fit? I had no idea what that was, but I nodded anyway. If Cal said I needed one, I probably did.

I was once again surprised by the amount of support that I was able to receive when I expected the exact opposite. I was very quickly discovering that the community of people within the sport were extremely supportive and encouraging, and Cal was no different. In fact, it was his initial support that gave me the confidence to start looking into races and set a timeline to complete the Ironman.

In March 2013, when I began actively looking, there were a number of Ironman races in the circuit, some more popular than others. At that time, the popular races were prone to sell out within minutes of opening online. I learned very quickly that the popularity of the race was directly proportional to the logistical ease of getting to the race and the flatness of the course. For example, Ironman Arizona and Ironman Florida, both very flat and very easy to get to, sell out within minutes of opening. As a result of the popularity, qualifying for Kona at one of these races required a near professional performance. Winners of a competitive age group often finish in under nine hours. On the other hand, Ironman Lake Tahoe, a race held at about seven thousand feet of elevation, far away from any major airport, and potentially colder than the proverbial witch's tit, never sold out. Consequently, the Kona qualifying times were closer to, and often above, ten hours.

I quickly became intrigued by an Ironman that checked a lot of the boxes of the latter example. It was a race that was a bit challenging to get to and with difficult conditions—nearly six thousand feet of elevation gain over rolling terrain on the bike. Also, it was expected to top ninety degrees during the hottest part of the day. The race was Ironman Los Cabos, which was at the very tip of Baja, Mexico.

There was one other thing that entered my mind as I considered this race. During the last time I had been to Cabo San Lucas, I had gone there with the singular purpose of drinking my way through a vacation. I had succeeded in that mission during one of my darkest depths of depravity. I saw this particular race as an opportunity for redemption and to make amends to an entire city that I had completely disrespected. I now had a chance to show respect to an entire town and demonstrate to myself that I didn't need to drink on vacation to enjoy myself.

As Ironman Los Cabos appeared on my radar, the inaugural race was about to be held on March 17, 2013. This would give me the perfect opportunity to follow the race and see if it would be a good fit. From a logistical standpoint, it made a lot of sense. It was a cheap 2.5-hour flight from Orange County, and the climate was only slightly more extreme than San Clemente, where I lived.

I followed along with the blog and watched in wonder as the pros conquered the course in an epic fashion. The water was crystal clear, and the sun appeared hot, yet they all pressed through it. I was inspired again and thoroughly convinced that

I needed to go through with this race. I committed to becoming one of the finishers in 2014.

I registered for the race soon after it opened because I was convinced that a destination race in beautiful Cabo San Lucas would sell out quickly. Boy, was I wrong. The race ended up never selling out. There were likely a few reasons for this, but primarily it came down to the fact that the course was hot and challenging. Even people who are considered extremophiles often tend to seek the path of least resistance.

Upon clicking "Submit" on the entry form, my stomach dropped and I had an "Oh, shit!" moment. *What the hell did I just do?* I had never done a triathlon, never properly swam in the ocean, and now I was signed up for a fucking Ironman Triathlon in *Cabo San Lucas!* I officially had one year to become an Ironman triathlete.

Coke Fiend

IRONMAN VINEMAN, 2016. MILE 123.

The second I tasted it, I felt the warmth in my bloodstream, reminiscent of my first sip of alcohol, but it was immediately followed by an opposing sensation: a sudden burst of energy and hyperawareness, which was new to me. My pain was diminished just enough to let me hold pace.

I felt unstoppable, invincible, unbeatable, all thanks to my wonderful new drug:

Cola.

Of course, I had tasted cola before. In fact, it was an almost daily dietary staple in my previous life. I enjoyed it, maybe even a little too much. I had never, however, tasted cola during an Ironman marathon. Now, I was officially woke.

I had never thought of cola as much more than a delicious beverage that happened to rot our teeth and give us diabetes.

Now, I understood. Cola was divinely inspired, intended for the gods to harness as nectar for their strength and immortality. In the hands of humans, it could be a destructive or empowering force. Death for the sedentary, but rocket fuel for the champions, gifted to mortals by Zeus himself, to be delivered in a Dixie cup at mile eight of an Ironman.

I then felt a little sadness that it had taken me five Ironman Triathlons to discover cola as "nutrition" for a race. Up to this point, when I ran through an aid station, I went straight for Gatorade and water, thinking cola was reserved for the poor, desperate souls trying to grasp at anything to keep them going. It was a last resort.

Those were the conditions that led me to take the fizzy brown liquid from the nice lady in the orange volunteer shirt. I was feeling the hurt, and the thought of eighteen more miles of Gatorade made me want to vomit. I stumbled through this aid station, thinking I would be spending another marathon walking, until I tasted the perfectly sweet beverage and felt my legs come to life.

The sensations that hit my synapses were a not-so-gentle reminder that, indeed, I am an addict. I immediately wanted more.

I trotted off with a newfound motivation to make it to the next aid station to get my next fix. It was a shallow motivation, but one that kept me going. Whether the effect was purely psychological or chemical, I can't be sure, but there's no doubt that my spirits were higher, and I was now able to tap into a greater physical capacity that I had not yet known I had.

"Trust your training," I had always heard, yet up until this point, I was unable to fully replicate the training paces during a race. Finally, after getting a hit of cola, I was running *faster* than I had in training. I was finally tapping into the full potential my training had allowed.

8

TRAINING DAY

S tep 1: I had to buy a bike trainer.

It had been a few weeks since my surgery, and I could finally keep my arm out of a sling for most of the day. The doctor's orders were to avoid running for a few more weeks, and I couldn't swim for a couple more months. My big problem was that the clock was ticking for my road to Ironman Los Cabos. I had just under a year to be ready to swim, bike, and run 140.6 miles, and I could do exactly none of those things for any fraction of that distance.

I could walk, and I could finally ride a stationary bike. That's where I began.

Let me be clear that I had never owned a road bike, nor had I ridden one. The bike I owned was the same cheapo mountain bike I had bought and used only once before being shamed for having the audacity to try to ride it out in the open. The drive-train was now rusty; there was still nine-year-old mud caked in the nooks and crannies, and the welded seams were clearly visible where each tube met its counterpart. It weighed around forty pounds, and every single moving part squeaked, crunched, creaked, or clanked.

I enthusiastically removed it from its hiding place in our garage, dusted off the spider webs, and secured it to a brand new $90 bike trainer I had bought online. I didn't bother pumping up the tires because (a) I didn't have a bike pump, and (b) I hadn't removed any air from the tires so logic would dictate that air would still be in them. I would make about a trillion and sixty-five more errors in judgment throughout the course of the next year as a beginner triathlete.

I took a step back from the mounted bicycle and took a deep breath.

Day one of Ironman training, I thought to myself.

I needed motivation for this. I couldn't fathom the idea of staring at a blank wall for thirty minutes. I needed some entertainment. I opened YouTube on my tablet and searched for "Hawaii Ironman." Hundreds of results came up. I began playing the first one, which was the 2011 edition of the Ironman World Championship. I was introduced to Craig Alexander and Chrissie Wellington. Apparently, Wellington had been a dark horse coming into Ironman, but she proceeded to win every single freaking race that she entered. Her badassness was veiled by an "aw, shucks" kind of humility.

Maybe I have some kind of hidden talent like Chrissie Welling-ton, waiting to be unleashed on the world, I thought to myself.

I tightened up my twenty-dollar ultra-white Marshall's tennis shoes, officially accessorizing my "dad bod," and mounted ol' Rusty. I began pedaling and was amazed by how easy it was. I was barely breaking a sweat. Maybe this triathlon thing wouldn't be so hard after all.

I shifted up to a harder gear, and it still felt ridiculously easy. I shifted up again, and again, and again, each time, the expected increase in resistance did not come.

I was now in the hardest gear, and the workout still felt effortless. I brought my ego back to reality. I was not some closeted amazing athlete who could jump onto a trainer and start grinding easily away at four hundred to five hundred watts. Something must be wrong.

I looked at the rear wheel and immediately realized that it was simply floating in the air with no flywheel attached to provide any sort of resistance. It was as if I was Elliot flying through the air with E.T., pedaling over a vast nothingness below me, only I didn't have a lovable extraterrestrial in a basket in front of me, and I was in my garage. It was a dumb oversight, and I wasted ten minutes.

Frustrated, I affixed the manual resistance flywheel to the rear bike wheel and got back on the bike.

Take two.

I mashed my feet down on the pedals as if I were stepping into deep, thick piles of mud. The years of caked rust and dirt were breaking free as I continued to press down on the pedals. As the wheel gained momentum and the crud broke free, the pedaling became easier, but a loud, constant noise grew from the rear tire. It sounded like a leaf blower was coming out of my ass.

The combination of low tire pressure and notched mountain bike tires created a deafening sound against the flywheel, which probably caused the neighbors to wonder what mad scientist project I was working on in my garage. But they weren't hearing a science project at all. They just heard some idiot, who was the only person on planet Earth who had ever attached a notched mountain bike tire to a trainer.

Meanwhile, I had my first opportunity to witness the effects of heart rate training. The results were discouraging to say the least. Now that I had some resistance on the tire, I was actually doing work, albeit very light work. Still, my heart rate reacted as if I were being chased by a pride of lions being chased by a pack of hyenas being chased by a herd of elephants.

My goal was to stay below 142 beats per minute. This was my "magic number." It was my result using Maffetone's calculation. I took 180 − 33 = 147. I then subtracted five more beats because I knew I was in terrible shape, and part of the instructions were to add a few points for good health and subtract a few for poor health. With a bum shoulder dangling off to the side and belly fat hanging over my sweatpants, I considered myself in the latter category.

I found very quickly that the task of remaining below 142 would be difficult because my heart rate immediately jumped above that number within about a minute of training with the slightest resistance. Despite my best efforts, my heart rate continued to creep up above 150, above 160, and nearly 170 before I stopped pedaling altogether to try to bring the heart rate back down. I could now feel my heart beating out of my chest. I became instantly aware of the fact that my body was not operating efficiently, and my aerobic fitness was, to put it mildly, lacking.

To be successful with the Maffetone Method, I had to slow it down. Clearly my body was conditioned to burn glycogen rather than fat as the primary source of fuel. My mind immediately questioned the legitimacy and efficacy of this training protocol. Was everything I read just a bunch of baloney? Hell, I wasn't even sure if it were physically possible for me to remain below 142 beats per minute with how things were going.

I owed it to myself to give it another try. I heard my sponsor's voice in my head relaying one of his many AA wisdom nuggets: "Don't leave before the miracle happens."

Having already experienced one miracle, I figured it was worthwhile to stick around for the next.

I scaled down the resistance a lot and began riding again. This time I only felt slightly more resistance than when I didn't have any resistance at all. I checked my heart rate. 130...135...137...

Okay, this was more like it. It didn't feel like much of a workout, equivalent to maybe a brisk walk, but at least my heart rate was cooperating. After a frustrating thirty minutes of stopping and starting to bring my heart rate back down below the magic number, and hearing the *Texas Chainsaw Massacre* going on behind me, I finished my first Ironman training workout.

As frustrating as the first workout was, I did notice something very remarkable. I felt fantastic. I felt energized. I felt clear-headed and motivated. I was so accustomed to feeling sore, beat-up, and exhausted from the workouts that I didn't think it was possible to feel so good from exercise. Maybe there was something to this easy training.

I immediately retired to my office to read up on aerobic fitness training a little more. If nothing else, it would ease my mind that I was doing it right. I also needed to research how to ride a bike trainer properly. It didn't take long to learn that a smooth tire is necessary to ride a trainer quietly. Also, it was advised not to buy cheap bike trainers, which I had done. Lesson learned. At least it was only temporary. As soon as I was able, I would be riding outside.

In order to ride outside, and ultimately race in an Ironman, I needed to bite the bullet and buy a bike that didn't sound like and weigh as much as the Clampetts' Oldsmobile from *The Beverly Hillbillies*. Clearly, Rusty was not going to cut it for the long term. There were a couple of reasons why I was hesitant to buy a new bike. First, bikes are very expensive. I could expect to spend a couple grand on an entry-level triathlon bike. Second, I was incredibly intimidated to walk into a bike shop and purchase one. My alcoholic brain and ever-present anxiety made me believe a bike shop owner would try to take advantage of me, criticize me, or make fun of me for stupid ideas (like racing an

Ironman with no experience). I was sure that the proprietors of a bike shop, rather than wanting to take my money, would instead find more delight in laughing at me for having such a silly desire to adopt a healthy new lifestyle. Welcome to irrational fear, everyone.

I decided to talk to a trusted resource first. Cal had been an incredible source of knowledge for all things triathlon in the weeks he had been my physical therapist. Being an avid cyclist, I figured he could be the one to point me in the direction of a new bike.

He recommended a bike shop in Dana Point, and I decided to check it out. I intended to save some money for a while before pulling the trigger on a new bike, but there was no harm in just looking, right?

I approached the bike shop as if I were entering an adult bookstore. I almost didn't want anyone to see me because of how ridiculous I felt going into a place where I didn't think I belonged. My apprehension calmed when I saw the bike promotion right at the entry to the shop. It was a package that seemed to be created just for me. It was an entry-level triathlon package, including a fully equipped triathlon bike, bike helmet, shoes, and a wetsuit for $2,000. I knew that all of these things, sold separately, would cost up to a thousand dollars more than that.

I stood next to the display, looking as though I was scrutinizing every aspect of the bike, when, in reality, I had absolutely no clue what I was looking at and was just trying to passively get the attention of a merchant to kindly rescue me from my ignorance.

I did know one thing. The particular bike brand featured in the promotion, Orbea, was the brand of bike Craig Alexander rode when he won the Ironman World Championship in 2011. Little did I know that pros change bike brands about as often as fashion models change clothes. Clearly sponsorships work because it sold me on the bike.

Finally, the kindly bike shop merchant wandered over to me. "How can we help you today?"

I wasn't prepared for this question. How *could* I be helped? How should I respond? "I want to buy this bike" would sound too forward. "I'm okay" would just leave me continuing to stand there like an idiot, staring at this thing I didn't understand. I decided to take a more honest approach.

"I'm a newbie to triathlon," I said. "And I'd like to know more about what gear I need."

With great enthusiasm for my newfound venture, the bike shop guy answered all my questions and delivered some much-needed expertise. My beliefs about this community were beginning to change as I discovered that more and more people were likely to be supportive and encouraging rather than arrogant and hostile.

I walked out of the bike shop that day the proud owner of a new Orbea triathlon bike and all the necessary equipment to get me started. Now the waiting game would continue until I was fully healed enough to actually ride on the road. Until then, ol' Rusty on the cheapo bike trainer would have to do.

With all the necessary equipment at the ready, there was still one other element I had to tie up. I needed a plan. At this point, I was just doing what I could based on what I knew, but at some point, in the very near future, I would have to develop a path to the Ironman finish line. I knew how I wanted to train, using the principles of the Maffetone Method, but I didn't know how to implement them with any sort of structure.

If I was going the coach route, I needed someone I could trust, but I was so new to the sport. How could I possibly know who to trust?

Before I could find a good coach, I had to determine what I wanted. I wanted to qualify for Kona. I wanted to do it by using the Maffetone Method. That meant finding the most effective coach of the Maffetone Method. Which led me to the question: who was Mark Allen's coach?

I typed "Mark Allen triathlon coach" into Google and looked at the results.

"MarkAllenCoaching" was the first result that come up.

I didn't expect that Mark Allen had actually *become* a triathlon coach after his triathlon career ended. I guess I just figured that he retired to a luxurious mansion on an island somewhere, living off of his triathlon riches (a belief that certified my ignorance). As a coach, I was sure he only took on the elite of the elite. He wouldn't pay attention to an insignificant dreamer like myself. I clicked on the link anyway. It wouldn't hurt to check.

"Sign Up Now," the button on the front of the page demanded.

Reading further, I learned that premium coaching packages could be bought for twenty-nine dollars per week, which included a custom plan and email access to Mark Allen and his coaching team.

This option checked off a few boxes for me. For one, it was a credible option (six-time world champion sits well on a resume). It was also pretty affordable for a coaching service. Finally, it satisfied my reclusive, introvert side. The last thing I needed was a type-A coach calling me every day to find out if I was pumped for the day's workouts. I wanted a plan and guidance when I asked for it, but mostly I wanted to be left alone until I had questions.

I clicked on the sign-up button and found myself beginning a questionnaire. I figured I would keep clicking through all of the free parts until it asked for a credit card, and then I would stop. Not being able to do any triathlon-specific training yet, it didn't make sense to sign up for a plan until I could.

"What is the date of your primary race?"

This was one of the first questions presented. I entered the date of March 30, 2014, into the form. The webpage immediately spit back an error.

"The date of the primary race must be less than six months away."

Well. Shit. It was still April, which meant that I had nearly a year until my primary race. The universe was missing no opportunity to force patience upon me. If I went with Mark Allen's training plan, which I wanted to do, I would have to wait until September to begin the actual plan.

At my level of infancy within triathlon (I still had yet to swim a lap in a pool or test my new triathlon bike), I felt like waiting until September to begin training for a March Ironman would be cutting it quite short. This may work for people who have already raced triathlons but not for an absolute beginner.

Trusting that Mr. Allen knew what he was doing in advising against Ironman training over six months before the race, I decided to explore some other options to build my experience over the course of the following months so that I would be prepared to begin the Ironman training when the time came.

Why not set my sights a little lower to get accustomed to racing and gain some experience? That's logical thinking, right?

I researched some races in my area and came up with something of a race schedule to help me build experience with progressively longer distances over the course of the year. Ultimately, the plan was to start with a sprint triathlon, then graduate to an Olympic-distance triathlon, then a half Ironman, and finally the big show in Cabo.

I signed up for my first race, the Carlsbad Triathlon, in mid-July, which was about three months away. As this was a sprint triathlon—approximately one kilometer of swimming, 15 miles of biking, and 3.1 miles of running—I planned on training for this race "uncoached," relying on resources I would find on the internet related to the Maffetone Method. I would employ the help of a training plan included in the back pages of a book called Be IronFit™ by Don and Melanie Fink, recommended to me by Cal. That would get me started down the path until I could attach myself to Mark Allen's Ironman plan.

It would also mean that while I wasn't training for an Ironman, I was training as if I were training for an Ironman. I would be training for a sprint triathlon, but I would be training for it in overkill mode to develop a strong base level of fitness.

Another book proved to be a tremendous resource to me as well, Phil Maffetone's The Big Book of Endurance Training and Racing. Having come from an AA background, I was attracted to any how-to book partially titled "Big Book." It didn't disappoint. It included not only Maffetone's training methods but also his diet advice, which was astonishingly simple and straightforward. It was a welcome departure from the overly complicated and failure-prone diet fads that many people promote. While it was a "Big Book," the contents could be easily summarized: eat clean, train easy, and get fast. Boom.

My first race was booked, and the plan beyond that first race was beginning to come together. After Carlsbad, I began training for a half-iron distance triathlon, the HITS Palm Springs 70.3, in early December. During that training build, I could do a couple other races to help build experience. If I created a training plan with Mark Allen Coaching in July for the 70.3 in December, I could more formally follow a plan and build the endurance necessary to complete a half Ironman. Then, right after the 70.3, I could begin another plan to build to the full Ironman, giving me a little over three months to prepare. It just might work.

My official first triathlon race season looked like this:

- Carlsbad Sprint Triathlon, July 2013
- Semper Fi Sprint Triathlon on Camp Pendleton, August 2013
- Long Beach Sprint Triathlon, September 2013
- Oceanside Olympic Triathlon, October 2013
- HITS Palm Springs 70.3, December 2013
- Ironman Los Cabos, March 2014

With my schedule in place, my plan set, and my shoulder finally healed enough to endure the swim, bike, and run training, I was all set to begin. I was enthusiastic and ecstatic to start. The weeks of waiting, healing, and climbing up the walls were finally over. I was like a dog being let outside on the first day of spring.

But I had to remember the plan: stick to the heart rate.

As I began to venture out on workouts in the great outdoors, I experienced how difficult this actually was. I could barely maintain a run without my heart rate jumping to well above 142. I thought I was having a hard time keeping the heart rate down on the trainer, but that was nothing. I discovered that it was *easier* to keep the heart rate down on the trainer. Even cycling outside was more challenging from a heart rate perspective. This was exacerbated by the fact that riding outside required other elements of skill that were not required on the trainer, including balance, weight shifting, and "Oh shit" tension.

"Oh shit" tension is a term I use to describe the constant feeling of "Oh shit!" that comes with attaching ourselves to a high-performance bicycle and crouching in the precarious aero position. Aero position is relatively unique to triathlon, though it is also used in time trial bike racing. The aerobars extend off the front of the handlebars, allowing one to assume a more aerodynamic position. Unfortunately, there are no brakes on the aerobars, and the brakes on the handlebars, while only inches away, might as well be in another zip code. For a beginner, there is no easy way to get into aero. I just had to grit my teeth, clench my butt cheeks, and go for it. The resulting squirreliness causes "Oh shit" tension, and thus, heart rate increases even higher.

I spent the first few rides on my bike riding around my cul-de-sac. Scratch that. I spent the first few rides trying unsuccessfully to clip into and out of my pedals. Much like the act of a skier clipping into skis, a cyclist will often clip into the pedals of a bike. Combine that with the inherent difficulties of balancing on a bike, and the result is a recipe for extreme awkwardness and humiliating injury.

To the absolute delight of my neighbors, I repeatedly tried to clip into one pedal, followed by removing my remaining foot from the relative stability of terra firma, and then rolling forward in the hope that I could safely insert my free cleat into the remaining pedal. Once I found success with this, I had to contend with the other obvious hazard: stopping.

I'm sure that most of us understand the basic laws of physics and realize that a bicycle coming to a stop becomes increasingly more unstable. This means that there is a critical point at which one must remove a cleat from the pedal and place their foot on the ground to create stability. If this critical point is missed, a catastrophic embarrassment will likely occur.

This catastrophic embarrassment occurs for every beginner at least once. It is a rite of passage. In one day, it happened to me twice.

The mirth experienced by onlookers from this event is directly proportional to the humiliation felt by the victim. Within a matter of a couple seconds, a rider can go from looking as cool as a cucumber to spastically falling sideways like a vaudevillian comedian. It is a painful lesson, often resulting in a laceration on the shin where the gears of the bike's crank dig into the skin.

Each time I fell, I got up, brushed myself off, and tried again. Finally, after many attempts and near misses, I seemed to get the hang of clipping in and out. The next step was to become comfortable riding in the aero position. Continuing to put on a show for my neighbors, I chose to remain in the safety of my cul-de-sac until I could comfortably get into aero position and quickly get back to the brakes. Only then would I become comfortable enough to venture out into the great concrete yonder.

It didn't take long for me to get into aero effectively, but it did take quite a while to get *comfortable*. The challenge was mainly psychological. When one performs any activity that has an element of danger, the conventional wisdom suggests that "head first" is always a riskier and scarier proposition. This is true with water slides, football, headfirst luge (AKA, skeleton bobsled), bungee jumping, competitive wall smashing, and many other activities. It's also true of cycling. When in the aero position, a rider is putting their head as far forward and down as possible. The immediate impression this gives is that the rider will definitely faceplant at the next bump in the road.

When I was five years old, I rode a skateboard on my stomach for some reason. As I flew fearlessly down my driveway, I ran into a hose, at which point my face smashed into the concrete in much the same way as a *Looney Toons* character ran into a wall painted like a tunnel. Only my experience resulted in a fountain of blood spewing from my forehead and about four stitches, not a comical pancake face. It thoroughly freaked out my mom and ended my skateboarding career at an early age. Probably for the best.

So, yeah, head first on a bike was sketchy.

Further, being in aero made getting to the brakes exponentially more difficult. I would have to awkwardly move my hands, one at a time, to the handlebars and then squeeze the brakes. Not an easy thing to do for a beginner. In essence, while in aero, I had better be certain that there would be no reason to stop suddenly, or I had better become really good at getting in and out of aero position. My goal was the latter, but that would take some time.

Running offered its own set of challenges. Many of my first few runs were actually aggressive walks, geared toward keeping my heart rate down. Had my heart always exploded into hyper speed when I went out on walks? I guess it did. That certainly explained why I was so quick to run out of breath. Only now was I noticing it because I was using the heart rate monitor.

It was an exercise in patience, acceptance, and faith. Patience because I had to rely on my governor, my heart rate, to keep my effort down when I wanted to run ahead at full speed. Acceptance because I had to live with my current limitations. Faith because I had to trust that my paces would improve given enough time and consistent effort.

But would they?

My thirteen-minute-per-mile shuffle was not nearly fast enough to be in the ranks of a Kona qualifier. If this heart rate stuff was all just a sham, I would be wasting hours and hours speed walking myself into last place, or worse, a DNF (did not finish).

Faith was my saving grace. I believed that I would improve by using the Maffetone Method and training consistently. Regardless of the results, I was sold on the Maffetone Method, and I was going to be disciplined and consistent with it.

My education early on was trial and error. I learned that hills were the enemy. At this early stage, I couldn't even walk up a hill without my heart rate spiking. I had to find flat ground. This was a challenge because my home was located at the very top of a hill. This made the beginnings of run workouts very fun, but the ending was painfully slow.

Within my neighborhood, I ran about a half mile flat loop, which was fine for short runs. It actually gave me an opportunity to meet some new friends. As I ran multiple times by people's houses, I learned that a couple of my neighbors were actually triathletes. They became fast friends and an educational resource.

For longer runs, I drove down to a flat location, usually by the beach, and ran there. With flat runs, I had more control over my pace and heart rate. I monitored improvements effectively this way, too. One of the side benefits of being injured and forced to walk for a couple months was that all the walking I did had kickstarted my aerobic training. While I struggled on the first few runs, my results began to improve dramatically after a couple weeks. This was the product of a very healthy diet, discipline, and consistency.

Once a month, I engaged in a maximum aerobic function (MAF) Test, a running test designed by Phil Maffetone to measure improvements under a constant heart rate. At the beginning of March, I did my first MAF test after just a couple weeks of run training. My results were three miles at well over a pace of eleven minutes per mile at a 142 heart rate. By April 1, my result was about a minute per mile faster. By May 1, my result was just over nine minutes per mile. The progress was stunning.

I was amazed and thoroughly optimistic. At this rate, I would be running a six-minute mile at an aerobic heart rate by the summertime. Look out, professional Ironman field!

Of course, this attitude came before I learned the demoralizing effects of the plateau. I arrived at a nine min/mile pace very quickly, but that's where I stayed. For the next few months, I varied between nine- and ten-minute miles, depending on the distance and intensity. Those early gains, however, lit a fire in me and gave me confidence that the program works. I was confident that in the right time, my fitness would continue to improve as long as I stayed consistent with my diet and workouts.

There was just one major element left that I had to contend with, and to me, it was the most challenging and frightening of them all: the swim.

Non-Wetsuit

IRONMAN TEXAS, 2015. MILE 0.1.

I can't breathe!

  There are too many people around me!

  I'm sinking!

All these thoughts rushed through my head during the first few hundred yards of every triathlon in which I had competed, but Ironman Texas had an additional challenge. It was a non-wetsuit swim.

To some people, this may seem like an insignificant variable, but to the adult-onset swimmer who believes himself to be about as buoyant as a Chevy Malibu, it's a game changer.

I knew that Ironman Texas was going to be a non-wetsuit swim. I had prepared for that reality by doing many open-water swims without a wetsuit, but it was difficult to prepare for the panic attack that inevitably occurs during an adrenaline-infused Ironman swim start.

The human body is not designed to jump into a large, disgusting body of water at seven o'clock in the morning. It's just not. I don't care what other people might say. Anybody who says it's refreshing is absolutely lying or brainwashed. The overwhelming shock of the body realizing "Oh, shit! I'm in a large disgusting body of water, and I'm being punched in the face repeatedly" is enough to cause a person to believe they are going to die a horrible death.

Hence my present situation. I was no more than two hundred yards into Ironman Texas, in front of hundreds of rowdy spectators, and in the midst of a panic attack. I swam off to the side of the crowds of overenthusiastic swimmers and rolled over onto my back in an attempt to float, but the turbulence of the water kept forcing chops of water over my mouth and nose.

If I had a wetsuit, I wouldn't have this problem, I thought to myself.

A neoprene wetsuit provides additional buoyancy, which for a nervous swimmer is very welcome in an open-water swim. Added buoyancy also means less energy is exerted to stay afloat, and thus faster movement through the water. In this race, because the temperature of the water was too high, wetsuits were not allowed.

I felt like I was sinking, my heart was racing, and I couldn't catch my breath. All this and I still had 140 more miles to go.

All this because I didn't have a wetsuit. All this because I had an irrational fear of drowning in a race where nobody had ever drowned.

Leading up to race day, I knew this would be an issue, so I kept reminding myself that this was a shallow water lake. If I got into trouble, I could just grab a kayak or, hell, even swim to the side of the lake and stand up. All of that went out the window when I actually started swimming and the enormity of my situation caught up with me.

I reminded myself that I had covered the distance many times in my training without a wetsuit, and I had done many open-water swims in the past and survived. This was my third Ironman, and I had proven I could do it before.

Perhaps it was the verbal reinforcement I had given myself. Perhaps it was the brief break that allowed me to catch my breath. Perhaps I just started out too fast. Or it could have been some combination of the three, but I was able to collect myself, and my confidence was regained. My ego was a little scarred, but I got over it and pressed on through the disgusting murky waters of Lake Woodlands.

9

GRACEFULLY
DROWNING

The box from Amazon was lightweight but heavy in my hands. The contents were an article of clothing I thought I would never wear again. It was a Speedo, and this time I was actually going to wear it out in the open.

As a poorly shaped man in my thirties, with more hair on my back than on my head, I had a lot of audacity donning a Speedo. The sight of me in budgie smugglers would be made all the more entertaining by the inevitable flailing about that was about to happen in the pool.

It was now May, and I was well into my "Be IronFit" training plan. I had consistently followed the plan and seen my running paces begin to drop ever so slightly from twelve to thirteen minutes per mile to about ten minutes per mile below my 142 magic heart rate within just a few weeks of running. I was having to stop and walk to bring my heart rate down less and less.

The cycling was beginning to come together also. I was able to ride outside on my fancy Orbea triathlon bike. Fortunately for me, Cal offered to give me a bike fitting for free. He was working on building his own experience as a fitter, so he saw it as a favor, and as did I. The bike fit made a dramatic improvement to my comfort, and I finally had the "Oh, I get it now" moment. I started to understand how a person could ride a bike for over five hours (though I wasn't nearly at that level yet).

One of the common things that frightens people away from the sport of triathlon is the idea of riding a bike for many hours. This fear stems from the idea that one's posterior could not possibly hold up for that period of time while sitting on a bike seat. That was certainly my fear after spending just thirty minutes at a time on ol' Rusty. The reality is that a proper bike fit fixes this issue. Properly fit, and with proper fitness, riding a bike for five hours is no more uncomfortable than riding in a car for five hours (still uncomfortable, but manageable).

I was making a ton of progress, but I still had yet to set foot in a pool. Finally, the doctor gave me the green light to begin swimming, just two months away from my first triathlon in which I would have to swim a kilometer in the open ocean.

Oddly, I didn't fear the swim itself as of yet. I had spent my entire life playing in the Pacific Ocean but never swimming out past the breakers. I didn't quite know what to fear yet. That would come later.

So there I was, holding up my first Speedo since high school. It was time to try it on.

Sure enough, I looked like Sasquatch in a tight pair of briefs. Lesson #462 for this beginner triathlete: I had to do something about my body hair.

I'll admit it. At that time in my life, I still subscribed to the toxic masculine paradigm that freshly shaved legs and chest were reserved for the less "manly" among us. There was nothing manlier than a hairy chest. Ask Magnum P.I., Burt Reynolds, or Austin Powers.

Staring at myself in a Speedo, looking as if I were in a poorly made sequel to *Teen Wolf*, I abandoned all of my prejudices and got hair clippers.

I didn't go to the razor immediately. That was just too sudden. I started with some clippers on the number one setting. I figured by doing that, I could ease into hairlessness. Going immediately to baby bottom smooth would surely result in looks of shock and horror to people who saw me. What I didn't realize was that zero fucks were actually given by anyone else as to whether or not I shaved my body.

I trimmed the forest, so to speak, and put the Speedo back on. It was slightly better, though my belly was still rolling over the tight elastic. Now it was time for the next scary step: to wear the Speedo in public at the local swimming pool. It's strange, but my intimidation wasn't necessarily related to swimming itself, but rather wearing skintight briefs while doing so. It was definitely outside of my comfort zone.

In the preceding weeks, I researched the best way to approach beginning swim training. I had no clue what I was doing, so I entertained the idea of getting a swim coach. Throughout my research, I kept running into a program called Total Immersion™. I learned about it first from a TED Talk by noted author, Tim Ferriss, and then from various triathlon forums around the internet. There seemed to be a hung jury on the program. Lifelong swimmers were, for the most part, critical of the program because it failed to address certain technical skills, while "adult-onset swimmers" who learned from the program praised it. That simple fact sold it for me. I'm naturally a contrarian and seeing that someone had developed a way for adults to learn how to swim effectively despite never having set foot in a pool was a welcome notion to me.

The idea around this program is to introduce people to swimming through a series of non-threatening progressive steps. First, it teaches us to glide in the water. Gradually, strokes are introduced, and finally, breathing. The breathing comes last because it's the most intimidating and challenging for people to grasp. If people learn to find their stroke rhythm first, breathing can be introduced more effectively at a later time.

I opted to buy the DVD, *Perpetual Motion Freestyle in 10 Lessons*, and started doing the lessons on a daily basis at the pool. I began to feel comfortable in the water with my Speedo, especially after I realized that absolutely nobody was looking at me with contempt or judgment.

Total Immersion was very effective, especially since I used it every day. Starting from scratch with the swimming, I didn't have a lot of time to prepare for a one-kilometer open-water swim. Getting in the pool every day was my way of cramming so that I could be ready in the shortest amount of time. The ridiculousness of my physical appearance was complemented by the silliness of the Total Immersion exercises. Exercise one instructed that I glide like Superman in the water by pushing off from a standing position with my hands in front of me and slipping through the water like a torpedo until my momentum was lost and my legs sank to the bottom. Then the process was repeated all the way across the pool. Those doing laps around me stayed out of my way in quiet annoyance and suspicion.

Yes, I was *that* guy.

Despite the silliness of it, I made rapid progress, soon adding strokes and then finally breathing. By the end of week two, I engaged in a practice that somewhat resembled swimming, albeit very slowly. By week three, I swam one hundred yards continuously, without stopping at the wall, in about two and a half minutes. This was a far cry from the flailing and drowning approach that my previous attempts at formal swimming resembled. In those experiences, I made it across the twenty-five yards of the pool, but only by sheer will, and by the time I got there, I was gasping for air.

By using the Total Immersion technique, the activity felt effortless and controlled. I breathed effectively. In fact, the only reason I felt the need to stop after 100 yards was because it sounded like a good round number.

After my third week of training with Total Immersion, I felt like it was a good time to start some structured swim training workouts. I pulled a few off the internet and decided to just start doing them at random, building up to about three thousand yards. Yes, it was a bit overkill, but I was training as if I were preparing for an Ironman. If I could go through a couple training builds before my first Ironman, I could have a better chance of qualifying for Kona.

The swim workouts were simple and straightforward, typically starting with a warm-up of a couple hundred yards, a few fifty-yard swims, and then a main set of a couple to a few hundred yards. Using the Total Immersion™ technique, I achieved all of these at a very slow, gliding pace. Gradually, my pace began to improve with increased efficiency and volume. By the middle of June, I rocked a hundred-yard pace of two minutes and ten seconds. If I sprinted, I got that pace down to one minute and fifty seconds. Michael Phelps would be quaking in his deck sandals.

Even though I was putting in a lot of focused effort in the pool and the work seemed to be paying off, there was one mountain I still had to climb before my first race. I had to do some swims in the open water.

Unlike pool swims, which are controlled, calm, and within a few meters of terra firma, the open water was unpredictable. In the ocean, there are waves, currents, and creatures, and this is all a considerable distance from dry land. A pool was the best place to learn to swim, but I had to throw myself in with the sharks...literally.

Even in my naïveté, I couldn't reasonably expect to have a nice, chill swim in a sprint triathlon without first practicing in the open water. That just doesn't happen. Let's consider what happens during a typical race start as an example.

A triathlon swim start begins either as a mass start (where everyone starts together), wave start (where predetermined groups of people start together in intervals), or rolling start (where people trickle into the water a few at a time in rapid succession). There is a common theme to varying degrees among the three. Many anonymous people charge aggressively into the water at the same time, fighting for a small amount of real estate in an environment where air is a limited resource. The potential for panic is very high and exponentially increases with every accidental gulp of water.

This wasn't necessarily a concern for me at the beginning. I think it was a defense mechanism to not acknowledge the soul-crushing fear. Yet, as the date of the event crept ever closer, the anxiety was beginning to grow. I had to get in front of the fear.

Thank God for the internet. Seriously. Thank God for it. I believe it was invented for introverts to look into local events, clubs, and activities without having to ask other people. It's a resource for the reclusive. In its vast electronic glow, I found a meetup for open-water swimmers that occurred every Saturday morning. The group swam around the buoys at Corona del Mar Beach in Orange County.

Swimming in a group is great. As an introvert, I don't necessarily have to interact with anyone. In fact, for most of the activity, it is literally impossible to talk with anyone else. The other people are simply there for support and a sense of comfort against the giant monsters lurking below. Though I do often wonder if a shark would look more fondly on a group of delicious triathletes rather than just one.

The idea of open-water swimming is actually pretty ludicrous. I mean, we're jumping into a deep, dark jungle of fear, where four-thousand-pound monsters with razor-sharp teeth lurk in the shadows, ready to remove our limbs at a moment's notice. Not only that, but we're dressing up as their favorite meal (sea lions) and flailing about as if we're injured. This is pretty much a death wish, and the only exhilaration that comes from it is surviving the activity and living to see another day.

I showed up to my first open-water swim meetup one cool, early July morning. It was a week before my first race, and I figured I could do one swim this weekend and one the following Saturday before the race. That would be enough to get the nerves out of my system. Thankfully, there were a few others who were newbies to triathlons, so I was able to find my tribe. From the shore, the swim didn't look at all threatening. The water was calm, and the buoys were laid out before us only a couple hundred yards off the shore.

In my mind, I was relieved to see how easy it looked.

This is nothing! I thought to myself. I mean, what was there really to be afraid of? There were gentle waters, a clear line of sight, and barely any distance to the safety of shore. This was going to be great!

As we approached the water and began to wade through the light shore break, the enormity of everything started to hit me. It was as if the buoys were getting farther away; the sea was getting rougher; and the monsters below, though they couldn't be seen, were ominously waiting in the wings.

"We'll all swim out and meet you at the first buoy," announced the leader of our group. Then he began swimming with grace.

I took a deep breath, dove in, and stroked with what I thought was an easy pace. The water was cold against my face, and I could feel the immediate instinct to gasp for air. This was much different than swimming in a warm pool.

I pressed on anyway and watched as the seafloor below me faded into murky darkness. Then the fatigue set in. I stopped and floated for a moment as I nearly hyperventilated. I became aware of my surroundings and saw that I was getting far from shore, but the buoy didn't seem any closer. People continued to swim by me. Even though I was wearing the equivalent of a full-body neoprene floaty device and buoyantly bobbing up and down in a saltwater bath, I felt like I could sink at any moment. I had an impulse to start booking it back to shore.

This is a panic attack, I thought to myself.

I had experienced panic attacks many times but not recently. I thought I was over them. I did all that work in sobriety to discover serenity, peace, and acceptance, yet here I was panicking because I stupidly thought I could conquer an Ironman without having ever swam more than a lap in a pool. *What the hell was I thinking? Was I really that much of an idiot? I could have lived a lovely life. I could have been sober, fat, and happy while I enjoyed my peanut M&Ms and cheeseburgers. But noooooo. I had to do an Ironman. Well, good job, Adam. Now you're going to die fifty yards off the shore of one of the calmest beaches in the world.*

Shut the fuck up, brain, I scolded, and then I took a deep breath...then another.

People underestimate the power of breathing, especially when in the midst of a panic attack. When we're full of stress, we subconsciously tighten everything up. Breathing becomes shallow, and anxiety increases. It's a downward spiral anxious folks know all too well. Yet we continue to neglect breathing and believe the story our brain keeps telling us that it's hopeless and we're in trouble.

The contrary action, to take deep breaths, is the simple and highly effective cure for this malady. All it takes is ten deep and full breaths. With each exhale, picture an area of tension (such as shoulders, neck, jaw, or hands) being completely released. Miraculously, the anxiety lessens. It's critically important to do all ten breaths because nothing happens for the first few. It takes a bit for the tension and stress to fully release, but it works.

I started to calm down as I bobbed up and down alone, even while the other swimmers faded from my view. I wasn't going to let one panic attack crush my dreams. I would take this challenge in chunks. My new goal was to swim to the first buoy. If I still felt like I was going to die, I could either swim back to shore or announce to the group that I feared for my life and needed rescue. While humiliating, both of these were viable worst-case scenarios, and neither of them would result in my death.

Taking the time to calm down, I discovered solutions rather than simply reacting to the problem. In the mind of an anxious person, the immediate reaction is that all is lost, but by breathing and taking the time to work through solutions, the person will find a better action than just reacting to the fear.

Additionally, the enormity of an obstacle can very easily be minimized by segmenting it into a series of steps. In the case of the open-water swim, instead of thinking of it as a full one-kilometer swim around a series of buoys, which caused anxiety over whether I could finish it, I viewed it as a segmented swim from buoy to buoy, all with the understanding that I was a short two-hundred-meter swim to shore. These are just a couple of the tools in my anxiety superhero utility belt. They don't take away the initial reaction of anxiety, but they do serve to squash the fear in its tracks.

I began to swim toward the buoy again, stopping a couple times to collect myself and take ten deep breaths. I made it to the buoy as the last swimmer, but I made it. Better than that, while still very anxious about my surroundings, I didn't feel the immediate need to execute one of the worst-case scenario options. I looked at the next buoy, which sat parallel to the shore from my current position. It was another couple hundred yards away. I decided I could try the same exercise. I would swim to that buoy, and if I felt like quitting, I could swim back to shore or ask for rescue.

I continued to repeat this process at each buoy until I no longer felt it was necessary. After a few hundred yards, I actually began to feel comfortable and started enjoying the swim. After about two kilometers of swimming, I returned to shore with some of the group.

I survived the panic of my first open-water swim and emerged free of any shark kisses. I felt like the king of the world. As I removed my wetsuit and began showering off with my fellow open-water swimmers, I felt totally comfortable in my Speedo. This was a far cry from the thirteen-year-old boy covered in a towel in the high school parking lot. Now, I wore it proudly. I earned it. It was a badge of honor for going to battle against the elements, and my own mind, and coming out victorious.

All of the elements came together a week before my first triathlon. The previous months had been spent slowly building my way up from nothing into to a cyclist, a runner, and now finally a swimmer. I fueled my body with the right types of foods, and my body was starting to resemble that of a triathlete.

The old me wouldn't have believed that this new me was possible. Yet so much work had gone into the transformation that the new me felt natural. I was comfortable in my own skin to the extent that the reverse was true. I couldn't fathom a life where I didn't come this far.

The test would come on race day.

I'm a Fish Now

IRONMAN VINEMAN, 2016. MILE 2.

This was the most enjoyable swim of my life. Everything about it felt right and good and comfortable. It was a river swim with almost no current and navigation was very easy. Since the river was relatively narrow, there really wasn't much risk of swimming too far off course.

At one point, near the swim turnaround, the river became so shallow that people could get up and walk if they wanted to. Many people did, but I chose not to, thinking it would ruin the integrity of the swim leg. Instead, I flailed forward like an awkward salamander next to a bunch of more highly evolved salamanders that had learned that bipedalism was a more effective way to get around in four inches of water.

Still, I made it to the last few hundred yards of the swim at Ironman Vineman feeling for the first time like I had actually had a good swim. In four other Ironman races, I battled fear before the swim, panic during the swim, and demoralization after the swim upon seeing my time, but I experienced none of these things during this race. I just felt the confidence of knowing that I was right where I belonged and doing exactly what I had trained to do.

There were many firsts for me in the swim leg of this race. For one, other swimmers were not passing me. It was not uncommon for me to be swam over by faster swimmers for most of the first half of the swim. This time, I kept up with many of the lead swimmers. Second, I was actually *passing* people. This experience was entirely new to me, and an empowering one at that.

Passing people gave me confidence to continue pushing the pace. I realized I was actually *good* at this swimming thing. My panic attacks disappeared and, thankfully, I avoided starting the bike race in the back of the pack. I finally raced with the leaders from the get-go.

I emerged at the shore and began the trot up the beach toward transition and caught my first glimpse of the time. The clock said 1:06.

My eyes widened, and I lost my breath, not just out of exhaustion, but also due to surprise. I couldn't believe that I just completed an Ironman swim time of one hour and six minutes!

Then, I realized that the clock time was not *my* official time and that I had started later than the cannon. I checked my watch and saw 1:03.

How the hell did I do that? I thought to myself. *I have absolutely no business swimming a 1:03!*

But, of course, it wasn't a lie. It was the result of tens of thousands of yards in the pool and open water, all with the goal of overcoming my self-inflicted limitations: swim anxiety and lack of confidence. For the first time, it had paid off, and I wasn't starting the race with a disadvantage. I was in this damn thing, and I was going to give these fast triathletes a run for their money.

10

IT'S A SPRINT, NOT A MARATHON

felt surprisingly calm on the morning of my first triathlon. I was eighteen months without a drink of alcohol. As a result of focusing my attention on transcending my inner demons, I was an entirely different person from the man who sat in a jail cell.

The man in the cell was two hundred pounds of anger, fear, depression, and shame. His blood was concentrated with alcohol, nicotine, and a variety of toxins from many years of self-inflicted physical and psychological abuse.

The man on the beach on this day was just shy of 160 pounds, confident, happy, and ready to dive into the ocean with hundreds of other athletes at the 2013 Carlsbad Triathlon. That man was me, relieved of my self-imposed shackles. I had a heart full of hope and optimism. I was the epitome of the "fake it 'til you make it" spirit within the triathlon world, living as if I were an elite triathlete, though I had never even completed a triathlon. Hell, I even shaved all my body hair. I looked like a genuine fucking triathlete, and I was no longer going to have to fake it. I was going to earn that title.

The relative calm I experienced that day on the beach was in stark contrast to the anxiety of the night before. It's important to note that an anxious person doing their first sprint triathlon prepares in very much the same way as a person who is about to undertake a year-long Antarctic expedition. I was no different. For this approximately ninety minute–race, I felt like I needed every accessory in the book along with backup accessories. Like a crazy person, I ran through every scenario in my head and overstuffed my transition bag.

It will be cold in the morning, so I better bring layers, I told myself. *It will be hot once I get started, so I should pack some sunscreen. How much water should I bring? Two or three bottles? Oh yeah! Electrolytes! Better bring a handful of salt tabs. Thirteen energy gels should be just about enough. What if my tire goes flat? Better bring a couple spare tubes. Oh, and a wrench kit in case I have a mechanical issue. And gloves! Don't forget the bike gloves! Wouldn't want to get blisters!*

It was as if my OCD had OCD.

Bringing my bike into T1, with a front hydration system, a bottle on the down tube, and a gear bag hanging off the saddle, I looked like I was preparing for a grand tour rather than a fifteen-mile, forty-five-minute bike ride. It's better to be overprepared than underprepared, despite how ridiculous it would make me look, and boy, did I look ridiculous.

While I looked like Inspector Gadget in a tri suit, my energy level was high, even though I hadn't slept much the night before. I learned pretty quickly that sleeplessness was a common theme for the night before every triathlon. In fact, one of the things I had learned from Mark Allen's coaching was that I had better get my sleep in two days before the race because the night before would be all tossing and turning.

After leaving my bike, along with a year's worth of provisions, safely behind in transition, a wave of calm fell over me. I walked over to the beach and stood amongst the other neoprene-clad racers and the anxiety turned into excitement. I turned my eyes upward and said thanks to God for transforming me and bringing me to this moment. I knew that every moment I was living free and sober was a moment of grace, regardless of the situation before me. Things could have been much different. *What if I had injured or killed someone in that accident? What if the accident had never happened at all?*

These opposing scenarios would have left me a prisoner. I would have destroyed a life, resulting in my freedom being deservedly taken away. Also, I may not have ever had a wake-up call to make a dramatic change. In both of these scenarios, I would continue to be a slave to alcohol and anxiety.

Instead, I was shown grace. While I could never look back on that incident with joy, I no longer had to look back on it with shame. I could be grateful for the grace it led to in my life. I wouldn't change what I learned and who I became for anything in the world.

As the age groupers started to line up on the beach and the gentle waves continued to build momentum and crash onto the starting line, things became quiet. It may have been because the anticipation was reaching a fever pitch, but in that quiet, there was a powerful energy hanging in the atmosphere, and it gave me an overwhelming confidence. It was a confidence I had discovered through training, but it was nearly lost a few weeks earlier on a training ride through my hometown.

Due to traffic congestion on Pacific Coast Highway in downtown San Clemente, bike traffic is diverted through the winding and rolling residential neighborhoods of the crowded beach area. Unfortunately, this diversion does little to relieve the safety issues that arise when bikes share the road with cars. Many cyclists blow right through stop signs and tear around blind corners while distracted drivers hunt for addresses or garage sales.

It was at a five-way intersection, and I was riding in the bike lane behind a car. After we both entered the intersection, the car took a late and unexpected right turn. The last thing I remember was seeing the PT Cruiser perpendicular to my direction of travel, which caused me to impulsively yell out in terror, "Holy fucking shit!" The impact caused me to fly over the handlebars, onto the hood of the car, and finally onto the ground.

It's an interesting realization to know what your last words will be. I always thought that if I died suddenly, I would do so in a PG fashion. Clearly, that's not the case. The rapidness to which my mind and mouth went to "Holy fucking shit" was astonishing. It's as if the phrase was sitting in a display case at the front of my brain, next to a small hammer and a sign that read, "Break glass when about to die." My brain had never been that quick to put words together.

There was no pain. There was no sound. Actually, there was a ringing in my ears as if a bomb had exploded next to me. I lay on the ground and watched as a number of onlookers came over to offer me help. Many also came over to look at the almost cartoonish Adam-sized dent I put in the side of a PT Cruiser.

While I was generally okay, and thankfully alive, I struggled to put weight on my left leg. After assessment, an ER doctor determined it was probably sprained. I was uncertain how this would affect my prospects for a triathlon in a few weeks. I knew at the very least that my confidence was shot. I had just learned to ride the bike, and now I had this new traumatic experience to shake my confidence.

The situation got worse. My brand new Orbea bike was destroyed beyond repair. If I wanted to continue with this sport, I would have to buy another bike. It was a decision that weighed heavily on me because the alternative would be to give up on my goal. I decided that there was no choice. I had to go forward. If I stopped moving forward when I hit a setback, I would always miss opportunities to grow. If I didn't get back on a bike soon, I would never get back on a bike again, and it would just become another negative reference point in my life. This sport was too good of a supplement to my sobriety to give up on it. I would not quit. I would not let something like a PT Cruiser stand in the way of my dreams (even if it could stand in the way of my physical body).

Because of my knee, I couldn't do any biking or running for about a week. This was four weeks before my first ever triathlon. Sacrificing a week of training and rebuilding my confidence on my bike so soon before my first race only added to the uncertainties of my new hobby. When I finally could start working out again, I started with super easy workouts so as not to further damage anything. This meant that all of my training leading up to my first sprint triathlon would be done in an easy aerobic training zone. Up to that point, I had done no speed or power-based workouts, and now I would not be able to do so before the race. Race day would be the first time I would "bring the pain."

By that time, I knew the value of patience. I trusted the process because I had enough evidence that it worked. But regaining my confidence was a bigger challenge. For a few rides, I was afraid of the same thing happening again, but as with anything, confidence is built with immersion. The more we deprive ourselves of discomfort, the softer and more susceptible to chronic fear we become. Therefore, it is essential to *always* seek out opportune discomfort. This is where growth happens. If we can't find potential for growth in discomfort, then we're just experiencing pain. By finding opportunity in discomfort and challenge, we become stronger. It is all in how we perceive that discomfort. A growth mindset is born when we become comfortable being uncomfortable.

By the time I reached race day, my bike confidence was fully regained; my knee felt fully healed, and my gratitude was intact. I was in the perfect condition to start a triathlon.

On the beach, my gratitude daydream was broken by the first air horn of the day, signaling the start of the race for the elite athletes. From my position up the beach, I saw a flurry of splashing in the shore break as the athletes dove under waves and battled for position. Gradually, they began to merge into a single file line of white water cutting toward the first turn buoy. As the beach emptied of the elite triathletes, the corral of age groupers began to move up the beach toward the start line.

Shit was getting real.

I could feel my heart rate race as I watched the second wave prepare to start. I wondered to myself if I were already in an anaerobic state since my heart was beating so hard. I took some deep breaths and continued to force myself into a state of gratitude.

The second air horn sounded.

We moved up the beach again, and I found myself staring down at the ocean. But something was wrong. There was nobody in front of me. I looked to my left and right and saw the intense faces of people who were here to race. The look on their faces said, "Greetings, fellow racer! I look forward to aggressively punching and kicking you in the face in a few short minutes! Have an enjoyable death by drowning at my hands!"

As a first timer who only had only a couple of ocean swims under his Speedo, and neither of them aggressive, I was definitely in the wrong position to start this race. I slowly started to inch back toward the rear of the wave. I looked around me again and saw the frightened faces of athletes that seemed to say, "Greetings, fellow racer! Please avoid punching or kicking me in the face in a few short minutes! I do not wish to die today!"

Ah, yes. This was my tribe.

As we waited for our turn to join the chaos, I enjoyed the brief moment of calm before the storm.

I don't remember the sound of the air horn that started my triathlon racing career. I do remember charging, err, shuffling toward the water well behind the aggressive swimmers. As I entered the water, a sizable wave approached us, and I watched as people braced for the impact. Instinctively, I did the opposite of most of the other racers and dove deep under the wave, emerging on the other side about five to ten yards in front of those who chose to brace for impact. This was the one area of swimming where I felt like I had an advantage. I spent so many years playing in the shore break that it felt like home to me. The heavy surf pounding the sand didn't scare me; it was the open ocean beyond it that always ignited fear within me. Now I found myself alone beyond the shore break, and I had nothing but open water between me and the lead group.

Bring on the discomfort, I thought to myself. I started swimming.

I followed a trail of bubbles, which came from the feet of the person in front of me. Every ten strokes, I looked up to make sure that I was on the right path and not swimming off to Catalina Island. A few minutes in, I caught a group of overconfident swimmers and had to dodge fists and feet for about a hundred yards toward the first turn. Once there, the congestion got worse as we had to navigate around the large red buoy. Once around it, the water opened up again, and I had the personal space to relax my stroke.

As I did this, I had a fantastic realization. *I wasn't panicking! I was doing it! I was swimming in a triathlon!*

At the very moment I acknowledged the fact that I wasn't panicking, the panic began to set in. It was a strange sensation of elation, followed immediately by a surge of discomfort in the pit of my stomach. My next thought was, *I should not be here.* That thought then escalated to, *I can't be here!* At that point, the intense compulsion to start swimming aggressively to shore kicked in. All of this within one millisecond.

Anxiety is such a fickle bitch. I stopped briefly in the water and looked up, partially hyperventilating, looking for a paddleboard or kayak to hold on to. Yet as quickly as it came, it left me as I realized that I had done this before. Heck, I was kicking ass in this swim. With my confidence restored, I pressed on.

After going around the final turn buoy, I headed for shore. The sound of the crowd grew louder with each stroke. Closer to shore, I was able to engage another talent of mine from my childhood: bodysurfing.

As I swam toward shore, I kept looking behind me to find the perfect wave, and I finally caught one to pass a few more people.

I exited the water, triumphant that the hardest part was over. Now all I had to do was ride my bike and hope I didn't crash. As I began to run up the beach, I experienced an odd sensation. My heart rate exploded, and I had to fight to find my breath. My legs felt like they weren't there at all. It was as if my brain was telling my legs, "Okay, let's go," and my legs were giving my brain the leg equivalent of the middle finger. When I finally did start to feel my legs, halfway up the beach, my calves started to burn and my feet clumsily trenched themselves into the soft sand with each step.

I didn't know it at the time, but exiting the water and immediately running toward transition is the single most energy-intensive part of the race. The act of going from a prone position to vertical forces the blood to divert itself from the upper body to the legs. Because the legs are far from the core and upper body, the rest of the body reacts quite oddly. One can become lightheaded, lactate can build in the extremities, and the heart rate increases substantially to pump blood to the farthest regions of the body.

Trudging through the deep sand with my calves on fire, I pushed through to the transition area and felt the sweet relief of concrete beneath my bare feet. I followed the crowd into transition and searched frantically for my bike. *Why the hell can't I find my bike?* Adrenaline, high heart rate, and the general rush I was in led me to forget where my bike was racked. I failed to anticipate that transition looks much different when it's full of bikes and people in the dark than it does when bikes have been removed, wetsuits are strewn all over the place, and chaos abounds in the light of day. Lesson learned.

Once I found my bike, I proceeded to overdress for the fifteen-mile bike ride. I put my cycling gloves on (unnecessary), four energy gels into my pockets (also unnecessary), donned my cool new shades (it wasn't sunny), and made sure that my two water bottles were secure (I drank no water on that ride). Finally, I put on my last accessory, a shit-eating grin, and left transition en route to the bike course. The photographer captured my triumph as I crested the hill out of transition.

The Maffetone Method taught me to hold back on the throttle during training, often to a painfully slow degree. Biking and running slowly is a tremendous challenge when the ego is shouting, "Go, motherfucker!" Through the formation of habit, patience became anchored in my psyche. The result was an obsessive focus on governing my effort, a significant competitive advantage in the world of type-A triathletes. It's also another tool for the anxiety superhero.

Often, anxiety and fear are products of a brain that leads someone to believe he needs everything right this moment. This is, of course, another great lie that the overactive brain tells us. Any positive result comes with time, and this requires patience and acceptance of the present state. Acceptance does not mean abandoning a goal because we are not yet where we want to be. It simply means acknowledging our current situation and accepting it as our present reality. Then, we make the efforts that we can from the present moment forward to move toward the result we want to achieve. Lack of patience and acceptance of the present situation leads to frustration, depression, and anxiety. For me, practicing the patient art of aerobic heart rate training forced me to accept my present situation, and consistent work rewarded me with tremendous fitness over time.

With months of patient practice behind me, the Carlsbad Triathlon was my first opportunity to put the hammer down and race my ass off. I tested my red line effort and saw how long I could maintain it.

Early in the bike ride, my mind told me that I would not be able to sustain such an elevated heart rate for a long period of time. For someone who trained in the 130 to 140 beats per minute range, finding my heart rate in the 160s and 170s was a bit disconcerting. The effort didn't feel terribly hard, but I could certainly tell that my breathing was labored and my heart rate was flying. To my delight, I held my pace quite nicely through the uneventful bike leg.

I climbed the hills and passed a few riders, and then was passed a few times myself. I was surprised by the seemingly sparse field of athletes. I remembered being cramped in transition amongst a few hundred other athletes and feeling concerned that I would be fighting for space. That wasn't the case. I found that we had plenty of room to ourselves.

Once I made the turnaround at the halfway point and started coming back toward transition, I began to see the crowds of athletes coming from the opposite direction. It was like a cartoonish dust cloud of triathletes all packed together. This was the first indication I had that I was actually doing pretty well. With that many people behind me, I had to be doing okay.

The confidence stayed with me all the way back to transition. As I approached the bike finish, I attempted to execute a seamless, non-stop dismount. It was an effort to look like a pro, and fortunately, I did not eat shit. For that, I was a winner.

This time in transition, I was focused on the task at hand. I found my gear without much effort, left my bike, put on my running shoes and race belt, and got out of there lightning fast. A perfect transition!

With one minor issue.

I ran out the wrong direction. I went toward the swim exit, not the run exit. As I trotted confidently back toward the ocean, a volunteer stopped me.

"Do you want to do the swim portion again?" she asked snarkily.

I considered this for a moment, confused by the question. *Why the hell would I want to do the swim again? Was this lady crazy? Should I just smile and nod?*

As if anticipating my confusion and next question, she quickly pointed in the opposite direction toward the run exit. Embarrassed, I performed a quick U-turn and exited out the correct way. Perfection doesn't exist in a triathlon.

I had done "brick" runs in the past, a workout where a run commences immediately following a bike ride, but in a race, it's an entirely different experience. The energy and effort are higher, and as a result, every little discomfort is magnified. Within the first two minutes of running, I felt my feet go numb.

That can't be good, I thought to myself but kept running anyway. I only had to run 3.1 miles, but without being able to feel my feet, that distance felt long. Numb feet aside, there was something magical about being able to run all by my lonesome, save for a few age groupers within striking distance. One of the benefits of triathlons is they attract about a tenth of the participation as running races do. I was turned off by running races because with ten thousand or more people at the starting line, it was nearly impossible throughout the whole race to find some open space. At the Carlsbad Triathlon, on the other hand, with less than a thousand athletes and a comfortable cushion due to the wave starts, I had all the room in the world.

Running off the bike is a really fun experience. Many people think that it is the craziest part. How could a person possibly run *after* riding their bike for so long? Simply put, we've warmed up, our legs are loose, and we can immediately get into a good pace if we manage our effort effectively. Running cold without a warm-up is not a very enjoyable process. It's only after the legs get nice and loose that the fun begins.

I was executing the run well. Off the bike, I felt great, aside from my numb feet. I was kicking off a mile pace that I hadn't achieved in my aerobic training, nearly a seven-minute mile. There were no side stitches and no gasping for breath. I was just calm and quick.

As I approached the finish line, I was right behind a person in my age group. He crossed the line, and I finished shortly behind him and heard my name called over the loudspeaker. I was overjoyed. Crossing a triathlon finish line immediately changed something in me. All of the training leading up to the race helped transform me into a healthy and happy human, but the act of finishing a race gave me *fulfillment*. Reaching the finish line allowed me to transcend my old self and find purpose.

Early in sobriety, I heard something profound from a man who was sober for a long time. Someone asked, "Will I ever get over my addiction to alcohol?" His response has stuck with me as one of the most influential statements I've ever heard about alcoholism.

He said, "As alcoholics, we have an 'ism,' and that never goes away. If I do it right, I never 'get over' being an addict/alcoholic, even if I never pick up another drink. But after putting enough days of sobriety together and working a program, one begins to experience a spiritual awakening, and that is a *transcendence* over alcoholism. Transcendence is not 'getting over' something. Transcendence means 'to rise above.' If we can rise above our addiction to alcohol, the desire to drink will leave us."

I didn't fully grasp that until I reflected on the race. Finishing that first race cemented my new obsession with triathlons. All the work and focus put into training, and ultimately crossing the finish line, allowed me to transcend my anxiety, depression, and addiction. It allowed me to live with a redefined purpose.

I rose above the broken man I used to be and was building a better version of myself.

I gave my new running pal a big hug, much to his surprise. I got the impression that he had done a few of these things before and didn't quite have the level of enthusiasm for finishing a triathlon that I did. It's tough to have boundaries at the finish line of a triathlon.

I became even more excited when I saw the results. I had finished in sixteenth place in my age group. That was in the top third. *The top third!* At one time in my life, I was the second-string benchwarmer to a bunch of stoned baseball players, and here I was, finishing in the top third of an endurance race. At that moment, in my own mind, I secured my credibility as a triathlete. I was ready to shift gears toward the next races on my schedule, which would ultimately lead to the full Ironman.

Going Dark

IRONMAN VINEMAN, 2016. MILE 130.

"Get moving!" the tall, muscular man in an American flag running kit screamed at me as he smacked my ass hard with his open hand. We were both running up Windsor River Road.

I grimaced in pain as the concussion of his hand to my ass reverberated up and down my body, causing my overworked muscles to tense and cramp. I only saw the back of the man's body after that, so he couldn't witness my reaction to his, um, "encouragement." Probably a good thing for both parties. If I can offer an obvious piece of advice to those reading this book, it's this: if you're ever on the second half of the marathon in an Ironman Triathlon and it suddenly enters your mind, "Hey! I should unexpectedly slap that person's posterior really fucking hard to support and encourage him as he runs up this beast of a hill," just don't.

Captain America's gesture snapped me back into the reality of my situation, a reality that is generally somewhere south of ugly at mile sixteen of an Ironman marathon. There were still ten miles left to run—not far in the grand scheme of an Ironman Triathlon, but to every single human on the planet, that's really fucking far. That is especially true to those in the middle of an Ironman marathon, where the body and mind are tested to the limit, and the only way to get through those ten miles is to shut the brain off and let the body take over.

I had been running pretty well so far, but it wasn't necessarily a sign that I was feeling well. I just knew how to *suffer* well. It was a belief rooted in stoicism, learned in the rooms of AA, and applied successfully to extreme endurance races. All human beings have to accept certain aspects of their present situation that are outside of their control while focusing intently on the things presently in their control. Many aspects out of their control are inherently shitty, such as feeling like junk at mile sixteen of a marathon. For some sadistic reason, the brain wants to focus on those shitty things outside of our control. There's only one thing to do about that. Accept it, and actively shift focus to the things within our control.

At this point in the race, there were very few things within my control. Primarily, I could put one foot in front of the other, drink water, and keep going. For the rest, I gradually accepted the present pain as a temporary and necessary path to glory. It was a way of shutting down my manic think-ing simply so I could operate the repetitive task at hand.

I was successful in keeping my brain out of my body's way until my new intimate friend decided to treat my ass like bongo drums. I walked for a brief moment, attempting to collect myself amidst the new and unreasonable hysteria occurring in my mind. I felt various levels of pain that were exacerbated by an immediate reaction to get my head back under control. It was as if all of the dogs were released from the pound at once, and the staff was frantically trying to catch them.

Who let the dogs out? Mr. Grabass.

A couple deep breaths and a slow steady walk sent my frantic brain back to the present. Once there, I affirmed to myself that I could keep running strong to the end despite the pain. A few moments earlier, I was doing just that, so why couldn't I do it again? A heavy slap on the ass shouldn't change anything. It was all in my head, and it was time for my brain to put all of the pain into the dark.

I once again focused on the simple and present tasks at hand: one foot in front of the other, breathe in and out, drink water, and keep going.

REBUILD

Transformation is an amazing thing. Regardless of how significant the personal growth, the bulk of the change occurs as a direct result of the first step. Within that first step lies all of the willingness, all of the pain, and all of the chopping away at the old self that creates a positive path forward. Beyond that critical first step, consistent action is necessary to avoid falling into complacency or back into bad habits.

It's like pushing a broken-down car onto the side of the road. Where is most of the effort exerted? Right at the beginning. It takes a giant push with your entire body on the car to initiate the first spark of motion. Once the car is moving, momentum is established and pushing the car becomes easier with consistent effort.

There's just one caveat. *We have to keep pushing the car.* Otherwise, it comes to a complete stop, and we have to repeat the difficult process again. This consistent effort is called *discipline.*

I don't want to confuse discipline with willpower. Willpower is an ability to "suffer" through some unpleasantness to produce a desired result. A person has willpower when they can stifle an urge to eat a donut for a diet. Discipline, on the other hand, is trained. It's a practice of consistent action in the direction of progress *no matter what.* A person practices discipline by establishing a healthy and sustainable nutrition plan and sticking to it every day, even though Janet is being a pain in the ass and keeps bringing donuts to work.

With willingness, we *start* pushing the car. With discipline, we keep pushing the car.

Throughout my previous attempts at sobriety, I had started pushing the car, so to speak. I established the momentum, but as soon as pushing the car became comfortable, I stopped pushing. Relapse ensued. As Arnold Schwarzenegger said to the children in *Kindergarten Cop,* I lacked discipline.

Triathlons, and more broadly, fitness and health, offered me additional strength and motivation to keep pushing. As I pushed, the desire to immerse myself in the joy and fulfillment of personal achievement led me to push even harder. It led to a desire to share my story openly so that perhaps other people might discover hope and gain the willingness to start pushing themselves.

After my first triathlon in Carlsbad, I felt validated in my ambition to complete an Ironman and chase the Ironman

World Championship dream. Before the race, I was certain that I could finish, but I still didn't know what to expect. Now, I had a point of reference.

Successive triathlons came and went during the summer and fall of 2013, and I grew from the experiences. I crashed hard on the bike portion of the Semper Fi Sprint Triathlon on Camp Pendleton near Oceanside, California, in August 2013. During the race, with automobile traffic on our left-hand side, there was a traffic-controlled hard left turn that crossed the road. About a hundred yards from the turn, a man driving a large truck thought he could get in front of the traffic and pulled out in front of me, causing me to swerve to the right to avoid hitting him. The turn came up quickly, and I found myself understeering it after the evasive maneuver. I knew I was screwed as I saw the curb approach with no chance of avoidance. I tried to slow as much as I could before hitting the curb. I went over my handlebars and faceplanted into the curb, getting road rash all over my face, shoulders, and arms. I don't know how I came out of it without any serious injuries, but miraculously, aside from a bruised ego and superficial scrapes, I was unscathed. Almost as important, my bike was okay, too.

Sitting in the ambulance, I tried to convince the EMTs that I could finish the race, but they strongly advised against it. The race official agreed with them and pulled the plug on my race. I was taken back to the race start and bandaged up by a few Marines in training. Upon exiting the medical tent, I looked like a mummy just released from his tomb with all of the excess bandages around my body.

While my ego and body were bruised, my resolve was still intact. I came back and finished the Long Beach Sprint Triathlon a month later and placed fifth in my age group. Then in my first Olympic, the Oceanside Triathlon, I finished seventh. At my first 70.3 (a half Iron distance triathlon), the HITS Palm Springs Triathlon, I again finished seventh. During every single race, I executed according to plan, and my confidence continued to build.

I spent the last few months of the year racing about every month, building up my endurance and the race distances. After HITS, which happened in early December, I didn't have another race until the big daddy at the end of March, Ironman Los Cabos.

I felt uneasy about the break from racing. It was an excellent opportunity to reset and begin a new training build to the race, but I was getting into a good racing rhythm, and I didn't want my confidence to suffer. This was the plan though, and I had to stick with it. The concept of periodization in endurance sports training is an important one. As we train for a race, we build, we peak, and then we taper. If we stay in a constant state of peak training, we risk burnout, plateau, injury, or a decrease in fitness. Through periodization, one gets the recovery necessary to adapt and build on fitness, thus getting the most out of every training cycle.

The three-and-a-half months to Ironman Los Cabos allowed me to have an effective training build without distraction or risk of burnout. During this time, I worked with Mark Allen Online, and his training programs worked well for me. Also, the encouragement from Allen and his team offered me the reassurance I needed to believe in myself.

Those months were filled with determination and drive, and my focus was solely on the Ironman finish line. I saw my aerobic running paces approach the low eight-minute mile for my long runs. My bike fitness was quickly becoming my strongest discipline as my longest rides approached six hours. I felt fitter, healthier, and more confident than I had ever felt in my life. Though my swim still left a lot to be desired, I had come a long way since the "Sasquatch in a Speedo" days. A four-thousand-yard swim was now a routine workout.

I also achieved another new milestone. I always thought about riding the forty miles to work on my bike, but I assumed it to be a crazy feat. Now, I was doing that ride once a week. This turned out to be a win on multiple counts because not only was it a healthy activity, it was an effective way to consolidate my time and get the training in. Typically, my commute to the office from San Clemente to Orange, California, took a little over an hour. Riding my bike, the forty miles took a little over two hours. Thus, instead of having to come home and do a two-hour workout at the end of the day or before work, I did my workout while I commuted and saved half the time.

These types of creative solutions gave me much needed experience in improving my productivity in other areas of my life. I learned time is not a static construct. Yes, we all have twenty-four hours in a day, but some people have figured out the secret of fitting more "time" in their hours. They just get more done, while others complain about "not having time." This is an excuse I had been guilty of using for years. I thought I was busier than everyone because I didn't have the time to do the things I wanted. The reality is that everyone is busy. Everyone fills each and every one of their twenty-four hours with something. It's just a matter of how one chooses to fill those hours and how effectively they use those hours.

It dawned on me as I began to fit nearly twenty hours per week of training into my so-called "busy" schedule that time is not static. Time is something that can be created at will. Once something turned into a priority, I made it work. It's a simple formula, really. Time is a product of energy and efficiency. Increasing one or both of these factors will increase the amount of time we have.

When I was energy-depleted due to poor health, I had less motivation to be productive. I performed tasks more slowly, made more mistakes, and generally accomplished less. When I became energy-rich due to healthier lifestyle choices, I became more determined, more creative, more powerful, and accomplished much more. Similarly, improving my efficiency through elimination, consolidation, or delegation dramatically increased the amount of time I had. Simple things like limiting social media time to a specific time during the day, preparing healthy meals for the week, or riding a bike to work were ways to make the most of my time.

Energy and efficiency also relate to one another. Without adequate energy, we lack creativity to discover new ways to become efficient. Alternatively, if we can increase our energy, we are constantly thinking of new ways to become more efficient and effective, which in turn provides more energy.

This is how top performers fit more life into their hours and accomplish more than others. It is a habit developed only through the experience of doing it. The only way we can start to do anything is to remove the toxic and false belief of "I don't have time."

The beautiful part about this equation is the role that aerobic fitness, especially in the form of triathlon training, plays in the results. Done right, exercise *creates* energy. It adds to our physical and mental capacity to do more in the time we have, but it is important that it is done correctly to be effective. Easy, aerobic exercise is the best way to maximize energy. Hard, anaerobic workouts consume energy and increase the chance for burnout over the long term, whereas aerobic workouts produce greater energy capacity. Aerobic workouts recharge and even expand our inner battery life, while anaerobic workouts deplete our battery.

I've had some of my best ideas and been my most productive during aerobic training. My motivation is increased; I tend to find solutions to problems I'm working through, and I have a clearer, more harmonious mental state. When this energy is created, I'm able to make so much more of my time. In reality, at least in my experience, training for fifteen to twenty hours per week did not become overwhelming, nor did it consume nearly as much time as I thought it would. Doing so only forced me to get real with how I was actually spending my time and forced me to create "quality" time.

Yes, fifteen to twenty hours per week exercising is extreme; there is no doubt about it. It's the equivalent of a part-time job. However, using lack of time as an excuse for not exercising is absurd. What sort of time commitment would it take to exercise for an hour every day? Seven hours is less than 5 percent of the total of all the time in a week. This leaves us with 95 percent of the week for everything else that we likely *don't* want to do. In the grand scheme of things, that's an easy 5 percent to find through a bit of optimization. Then once that 5 percent is found and used for exercise, watch how quickly the remaining 95 percent becomes more efficient.

One of the biggest apprehensions I had beginning my Ironman journey was the amount of time it would consume in my work and family life. I had visions of myself collapsing into a puddle of exhaustion in the middle of a crosswalk simply because all the training was pushing me over the edge. I found the opposite to be true. I was not falling asleep in crosswalks. Rather, I was becoming more productive, as if I were lubricating the gears of my brain to become more creative and resourceful.

Success with managing my time and making dramatic improvements in my quality of life came from a decision to commit. I burned the boats to the alternative options. I would not talk myself out of training. I would not talk myself into a jelly donut. I would not put myself down or practice half measures. I would give everything of myself consistently.

It paid off. I did every scheduled workout between December and March and progressed to the point where I was *theoretically* in the hunt for a Kona qualification. In other words, if everything went perfectly, I had a shot.

It was a long shot, but it was a shot nonetheless. Looking at the previous year's results of Ironman Los Cabos, I figured I would need a ten-hour Ironman just to be within striking distance of a Kona slot. If I could swim somewhere between 1:00 and 1:10, bike for a little over 5:00, and run a 3:30 marathon, a golden ticket to Kona could be mine. My training times put me right there, but would they translate in a race? That was the big unknown.

All I had was belief. I had never done the full distance before, and it would be the first time that I would race for longer than my longest training day. Even in the half Ironman, I finished at around five hours, which was an hour shy of my longest training day. At least during shorter races, I knew that I could continue without collapsing. The Ironman, on the other hand, was a different story. All the advice that I heard insisted that one does not need to train for the full amount of time of an Ironman to compete in an Ironman. In fact, it wasn't advisable at all to train for that long.

If that is the case, I often thought to myself, *then why is it advisable to race the full Ironman distance?*

Faith plays a much greater role in the Ironman distance than it does in any of the shorter triathlon distances. We have to have faith in our training to know that we've done enough to conquer the distance without ever having completed the distance. It's the ultimate test of how far the body can go.

That faith was strong in me ever since the day that I threw down the gauntlet and had the audacity to believe in myself. Belief was the first step toward achievement. It's a necessary step, but by no means sufficient to achieve a goal. Consistent action on that belief is critical, but even that isn't sufficient. With belief and action, we need adaptation or evolution. The definition of insanity is doing the same thing over and over again and expecting a different result. To avoid this trap, one needs to evolve and change the approach if something isn't working.

If I had continued down my traditional path of exercise and training, I would have burned out, just like I had dozens of times before. Instead, I researched and learned about the Maffetone Method, found somebody to model (Mark Allen), and made dramatic improvements off of the experience of those who had already succeeded.

In retrospect, it's easy to determine what I did right to achieve what I did. Having spent more than a year immersed in the world of sobriety and recovery, I was able to learn a lot about personal development and how to make healthy habits stick. The first element of transformation came down to an absolute burning desire to become something different. The desire had to burn so hot within me that the thought of not doing it would be too painful to bear.

When it came to sobriety, this was an easy association to make. Life as a drunk became so painful that it was too much for me to bear, even more so than the pain of living in fear and unfulfillment. That was the initial phase. Over the course of many months, I learned to associate so much joy with sobriety that the alternative of drinking was not even an option anymore. *Why would I go back to something so painful when I had this much joy?* The same process was used for triathlon training. Being an overweight smoker who got winded walking up a flight of stairs and was afraid of his own shadow was painful, yet so was exercise (in my perception at the time). Then I discovered a burning desire in me to complete an Ironman Triathlon, something which would give me tremendous fulfillment. When I found a joyful and fulfilling method of exercise in meditative, aerobic triathlon training, a new habit was born that would replace the old unhealthy habits and abuse.

Which brings me to the second element of transformation: replacement. The old habit has to be replaced with a new healthy, productive, or empowering habit. We can't simply eliminate things and create a void. How often does that work? We have all experienced times we tried to quit something with sheer willpower, only to fail because we had nothing to replace the void left by the old habit. An alternative habit needs to be created with disciplined action. For the alcoholic, for example, the new habit may be attending AA meetings and becoming immersed in a culture of sobriety. The act of going to a meeting instead of having a drink imprints new habits as long as the first criteria, having a strong desire to quit, is met as well.

The third element is finding a person who has what we want who can teach us how to get there, whether through direct mentorship or behavior modeling. In the world of sobriety, this person is known as a sponsor. This should not only be someone who provides valuable insight and guidance, but someone trustworthy, who shares our values.

Within the triathlon world, the person I chose to learn from initially was Mark Allen. I used his services as a coach and followed his example consistently.

These tactics only work if we believe in ourselves fully, approach it with an attitude of patient optimism, and consistently take action toward the goal. It's the difference between a virtuous and a vicious cycle. In one, we ride all the way to glory, and the other leads to despair, resentment, or hopelessness.

For most of my life, I was an impatient optimist, meaning I fantasized about a bright future but become frustrated because that future was not my present reality. This caused my optimism to fade and be replaced by cynicism very quickly. The lack of immediate gratification led me to frustration and a lack of fulfillment. I didn't appreciate the journey, and I fostered resentment at every turn. It wasn't until I learned patience and acceptance that I learned to develop patient optimism in my life.

Patient optimism is the belief that, with the right set of actions, everything will work out in time. Putting my ego aside and practicing patience and optimism freed me to follow a more effective path, grounded in the reality of my present situation. The result was often failure, but it was failure I could learn from. The successes would bring gratitude and become platforms for higher achievement. With every new success, I leveled up.

Patient optimism, and the progress that I made as a result of unwavering belief in myself and a year of training, brought me to the shores of Los Cabos on March 30, 2014: the day of my first full Ironman Triathlon.

La Meta

IRONMAN LOS CABOS, 2014. MILE 140.5.

Just ahead of me, a young boy who must have been no more than three years old stuck his hand out in anticipation of my approach.

I trudged toward him, tired and in pain, but euphoric that I was finally about to finish this race. I weighed the options in my mind of whether I should actually high five this kid. He looked so excited to briefly slap my sweaty, disgusting hand caked in Gatorade and God knows what else, yet as harsh as it sounds, I was seriously considering avoiding the contact.

I mean, I was going to have to slightly bend down to hit his lower-than-waist-level outstretched hand and that would create a chain reaction of severe discomfort within my already very fragile body. At this point in the race, after running for twenty-six miles, on top of a 112-mile bike ride

🏊 🚴 🏃

and a 2.4-mile swim, any abrupt disruption of pace or body position could be disastrous and result in an embarrassing faceplant a mere one hundred yards from the finish line.

I decided to risk it and slapped the delighted boy's hand with such force that even my palm began to sting. I didn't see the boy's reaction as I was focused on a bigger goal—the Ironman finish line. For all I know, I may have broken the poor child's hand or given him some unknown sweat-borne disease compounded by the stank of five to six porta potties I had stopped at over the past four hours. Here's a life lesson from someone who knows: never high five a person just finishing an Ironman Triathlon unless there is a hot tub filled with hand sanitizer close by.

I turned onto Calle Ignacio Zaragoza, the street where the triathlon finish was located, and saw the finish line arches in the distance for the first time. At that moment, all the pain, sickness, and despair that I felt over those last ten miles of the race fell away, and I experienced a new burst of energy. I felt as though I was floating to the finish line.

I reached my right hand out to high five anyone who was willing to high five me. Nobody did. Likely because the finish line was sparse with spectators. Ironman Los Cabos did not have the throngs of crowds of other Ironman races. In fact, arriving at this finish line, it looked like I was arriving early to a party that hadn't started yet. Still, I felt like a million bucks when I finally hit the carpet and ascended my way up the ramp to the finish line arch.

I thought long and hard about what I would do when I crossed the finish line. It was an important moment, one that would be etched in my memory forever. The finish had to be memorable.

Should I jump? No way, too risky. I could barely walk, let alone jump. Should I stand there like Hercules and flex my muscles? Nah, too arrogant. Besides, flexing my skinny arms would be laughable. How about a fist pump and a shout? Yeah! That's the ticket! My finish-line moment was set.

I failed to anticipate the effect that the ten-and-a-half hours of heavy breathing would have on my vocal cords. The run past the finish line and fist pump went according to plan, but the shout came out sounding something like a sea lion getting hit in the stomach with a baseball bat. It was more of a low labored groan than a shout, but it was the sound of victory, nonetheless.

The awkward silence that floated in the air after my audible clumsiness was fortunately broken by the announcer's voice over the loudspeaker. "Adam Hill from San Clemente, California," the voice said. "You are an Ironman!"

They were the words I had longed to hear for over a year, and they were a symbolic exclamation point on the journey from an alcoholic, unhealthy smoker on the fast track to death to racing among and being one of the fittest people in the world.

My feelings as I was corralled through the finisher area were mixed. I was overjoyed but in so much pain. I was exhausted but full of energy. I was hungry, but I did not want to eat anything. I was thirsty, but I did not want to drink anything. I was hot, but I was shivering uncontrollably. I was a full-blown contradiction, and it was tremendously uncomfortable, but I had never felt more fulfilled than in that very moment.

As I sat among the rest of the finishers, I thought about what would come next. Some would call it quits and go back to a comfortable life. I, on the other hand, was already plotting my strategy for my next Ironman to take place a few months later.

TEN PERCENT

had done it. I had become an Ironman triathlete. Not only did I achieve my goal of finishing an Ironman barely a year into the sport, but I was within the top 20 percent of finishers. My time was 10:45, well below the seventeen-hour cutoff, and just before the setting of the sun. Achieving the goal of finishing an Ironman, while a dream come true, was only the first step toward my ultimate goal of qualifying for the Ironman World Championship. To do that, I had to cut my finish time by nearly an hour. I had to get 10 percent better.

Ten percent sounds so simple. Just reach a little further, fight a little harder, give a little more. The final 10 percent is the hardest one could ever achieve, and every single percentage point within that 10 percent is progressively harder than the last. To become an hour faster at Ironman racing, I would have to become even more disciplined, creative, and adaptive.

In the two years after Ironman Los Cabos, I chipped away at that 10 percent systematically, slowly catching up to the leaders in my age group. Primarily, it was thanks to consistent and disciplined work with the Maffetone Method, a clean diet, and belief in myself. Plus, I had a point of reference that I could tap into to reinforce this belief: sobriety. Becoming sober was something I never thought I could achieve, but I did it through disciplined effort and willingness. Having sobriety as a point of reference, I knew I could achieve anything else I put disciplined effort toward.

I had gone from finishing between fifteenth and twenty-fifth place to consistently finishing in the top ten. Between 2014 and 2016, I completed four Ironman Triathlons and many shorter distance races, and I steadily improved my times. I was now chasing a psychological barrier of breaking ten hours in an Ironman, but I really needed to improve on my ability to swim effectively and run well off the bike to do so. My cycling ability was solid, and I was now consistently breaking five hours on the 112-mile bike portion. Somehow, despite my lack of experience in the discipline, I became a very strong cyclist and was getting used to coming out of the swim in the middle of the pack, only to pass hundreds of people within the first half of the bike course. Then, on the run, I could hang on for a while, but I would ultimately fall apart at mile eighteen and never catch the top guys in my age group. I ran a high three-hour or low four-hour marathon, but I needed a low three-hour marathon to win a Kona slot. It was a tall order to say the least.

Patient optimism and consistent disciplined effort paid off. At my fifth Ironman, Ironman Vineman in 2016, I broke ten hours for the first time and placed sixth in my age group, missing a Kona slot by two places. At a typical award ceremony, Kona slots are given out to each age group, and if any slots are declined, they roll down to the next place finisher in the age group. It's not often that a slot is declined, but I was still hopeful that a couple of athletes would decline, and I could punch my ticket. It was the first award ceremony that I actually felt like I had a conceivable chance of getting a roll down slot, but alas, it wasn't meant to be on that occasion.

At Ironman Arizona a few months later, I had a personal best race. I finished in 9:28. It was there that I finally felt my run had come together. I ran a 3:20 marathon off the bike and finished seventh in my age group, breaking the top ten in one of the most competitive Ironman races on the circuit.

I was right there. I knew I had it in me to qualify. I just had to train more effectively. I knew there were still missing pieces. In my investigation into what they were, I realized that I was highly effective and structured in my aerobic training, but I had very little structure in the anaerobic or "speed" training. I hated speed work. I hated how it made me feel. I hated how much it hurt. I hated how I wanted to puke after every hard interval. Because of that, I limited the speed and power at which I would perform them. I knew that if there were any variable I could improve, it was the speed work.

Within an Ironman training build, aerobic training accounts for about 90 percent of the total training load. Speed and power work should account for about 10 percent. The benefit of the speed work is not just to build speed (though that can be a benefit); it is primarily to provide the strength to endure late in the race and to develop the psychological fortitude to withstand the suffering that will inevitably come in those late hours of the race.

I was hesitant to engage in too much anaerobic work because my past was littered with attempts to exercise hard, only to get injured or burned out. The difference now was that I had a strong base of aerobic fitness on which to develop power and speed. As the analogy goes, before building a house, build a solid foundation. A house built on sand will not stand. Now that I had that strong foundation, I could build a bigger house. I could withstand more intensity.

I decided to revisit my target paces and power during intervals. This would require some aggressive estimating to find the best training paces. Instead of just going as hard as I could for the interval and falling apart halfway through, I had to target a pace that would allow me to be most effective. Having run a 3:20 personal best marathon off of the bike, I figured I could probably run an open marathon in a little under 3:00. Using a simple running pace formula for intervals, I determined my target threshold pace (for intervals of six to ten minutes) should be 6:30 minutes per mile. That was about thirty seconds faster than I had been trying to run them.

This was going to be fun.

As far as my bike power was concerned, it was time for more disciplined, power-based training on the bike trainer. Riding a bike outside is a lot of fun. Riding a bike on an indoor trainer is not so much fun. It does, however, do wonders for bike fitness. For one thing, training on an indoor bike offers a greater degree of control. There are no stop signs or lights; flat tires are not an issue, and it's about a million times safer because cars are not driving at 100 mph right next to me in my garage. Instead of having to worry about Mr. BMW swerving all over the road, distracted by his cell phone, I can set the power target and then grind away, relatively worry free. Aside from all that, it's boring as shit.

To start, I needed to do a functional threshold power (FTP) test. The FTP is the power that can, theoretically, be held for one hour if the expectation is to drop dead right at the end of that hour. Essentially, it's a twenty-minute, all-out effort where the resulting average power is adjusted to give an FTP result. After a painful yet heroic effort, my FTP came out to 275 watts. With this number, a whole new world was opened up to me. From there on out, I could establish training plans on target power.

With all of this effort to find that 10 percent improvement, I knew there was also another next step in my development. From what I had learned in sobriety, I knew that the next step was giving away what I had. I wanted to extend the knowledge and passion that I had gained to other people, specifically those who may have struggled with anxiety, depression, addiction, or unhealthy habits. I wanted to give them a simple and enjoyable path toward health and wellness. Extra Life Fitness was born.

My new journey required me to open up about my story. With a few years sober and a few Ironmans under my belt, I became an open book. In early sobriety, especially within the rooms of AA, anonymity is a key element. Hell, it's in the name. Newly sober people, including myself, struggle with shame, pride, and ego while we do the work to heal ourselves. Having a safe place that honors their privacy is a key to that healing, and it was certainly important to the security of my early sobriety. Many people wish to maintain that anonymity, which works well for them.

As I evolved through my own sobriety and discovered new life beyond the bottle, I found an alternate path to anonymity. Anonymity, for me, became a safety net and a comfort zone, which lacked a key element that was important to my long-term health and sobriety. It was an element that I had discovered through triathlons that helped me progress to the elite level I had achieved. That element is accountability. While I was accountable to my sponsor in early sobriety, I felt that the next phase of my development required an evolution beyond anonymity. Being forthcoming about my story meant I was accountable to my sobriety, health, and fitness.

Years earlier, before I ever understood this, I decided to abandon anonymity and shout my experience, strength, and hope from the rooftops. I felt it was the best way for me to serve others who may be struggling with anxiety, depression, or addiction. I learned later that this process of total transparency held me accountable, fortified the habits that kept me healthy and sober, and kept me on track and on the path toward life. I can't recommend this path to everyone, but it is important for everyone to understand how they are best held accountable, whether it be among a few trusted friends or shouting from the rooftops.

After training with Mark Allen Coaching for about a year, I received word that he was dissolving his coaching company. One of the coaches spun off a different company, and I was shuffled into that program for a period of time. After a couple years, I made the decision to forge my own path. In 2016, I became certified as an Ironman coach in the first year certification was offered, and began coaching myself. Within that first year as a coach, I also brought on a few athletes.

It was one thing to be accountable to my own progress as an athlete, but to hold another athlete accountable and have responsibility over planning their progression was another thing entirely. Honestly, it scared me a little. The nagging questions began to infiltrate my mind.

What if an athlete gets injured?

What if they train hard and fail?

What if I suck as a coach?

People depended on me to help guide them toward their goals. On one hand, it was scary. I felt the burden of their success on my shoulders. On the other hand, I was helping people to succeed in their passions, and that was incredibly rewarding. Life as a coach also offered me an opportunity to hold myself accountable. If I wanted to be an authority on the subject, I had to be exceptional at my craft. I sought continuous improvement of my own performance and experimented on myself to find the best conventional and nonconventional approaches to training.

For example, I learned a lot about breathing, both in and out of exercise. While breathing may seem like a conventional practice, I was exposed to a few nonconventional techniques to maximize the effectiveness of my breathing. My first introduction to the importance of breathing came from an eccentric Dutch man by the name of Wim Hof. Known as "The Iceman," he is famous for his ability to withstand ice cold temperatures for ridiculously long periods of time, and his interesting breathing method is touted as having some amazing effects on the body and mind.

I was attracted to his techniques after hearing the praises of people I admired, namely Tim Ferriss and Tony Robbins. The techniques themselves had a very low barrier to entry, meaning I didn't have to buy any equipment or invest a ton of time into mastering a technique. I simply had to follow a set of instructions and just breathe. Essentially, I had nothing to lose except a small amount of my time.

Hof has two primary elements to his training: cold immersion and breathwork. With the breathing technique, one does three to four rounds of forty deep breaths in and out followed by a breath hold off of an exhale (meaning the lungs are empty on the breath hold). Just the thought of holding my breath without any air in my lungs was enough to give me a panic attack, but surprisingly, after a round of deep breaths, holding my breath was easy, and I discovered quickly that I could surpass two minutes on a breath hold. Additionally, I found that my energy and serenity improved immediately. I've never found a simpler and more effective way to immediately improve energy and mood than this method.

Breathing during exercise also began to play a role in my training. After learning about how important, but ignored, breathing is for most people, I found that focusing on it could immediately improve performance. I concentrated on finding a breathing rhythm during workouts that effectively oxygenated my blood on an inhale and removed toxins on the exhale. I was also able to easily determine my effort level just by my breathing rate. For example, during a run, if I was breathing at a rate of four steps for every breath in and four steps for every breath out, my effort was easy. Three to one was a tempo effort, and two to one was a hard effort. It was an additional biofeedback mechanism to help me improve both aerobically and anaerobically.

It's amazing to me how breathing, something essential to living, is ignored by nearly everybody. Because it is involuntary and done at all times, it's taken for granted. For that reason, many people tend to breathe too shallow or too fast. For someone like me, a person highly susceptible to anxiety, shallow or fast breathing exacerbates problems. Consciously focusing on my breathing gave me yet another tool to manage my anxiety. Taking slow, deep breaths in a steady rhythm stopped anxiety in its tracks. An exercise I began to use regularly is ridiculously simple, and only takes a couple minutes to practice. Take a slow deep breath in for four seconds. Hold it for eight seconds, and then breathe out fully for seven seconds. After about five to ten of these breaths, anxiety will diminish.

By early 2017, my life had dramatically transformed. I had transcended the desire to drink. I was so enveloped in a new and healthy lifestyle that alcohol was no longer even on my radar, though I still had to constantly be on my guard (such is the life of an alcoholic). I discovered a world of sobriety within triathlons; there were many people who had found the spiritual purpose that I had through endurance sport. I wished I could shout from the rooftops what I had found and deliver to other people suffering with alcoholism the message that there is hope beyond the bottle and beyond fear.

Earlier that year, I was introduced to an interesting opportunity. My wife and I saw a casting call on Facebook for a new show being developed by NBC and Ironman. The show was to be called *Ironman: Quest for Kona*. It would feature ten athletes of varying abilities and demographics all trying to achieve one goal: qualify for the Ironman World Championships in Hawaii. It was a serendipitous idea, one that the patient optimist in me recognized as an excellent opportunity.

"How funny would it be if we tried out for this?" I asked my wife.

"I think you should do it," she replied in a heartbeat.

That weekend, I scripted a video introducing myself and my history. *How could I possibly fit my story into a one-minute video?* I thought of slow-motion close-ups of my face, capturing the intensity as I stared off into the void beyond the camera, sweat pouring down my face, muscles glistening in the filtered blue light of a darkened workout dungeon while "Eye of the Tiger" played in the background.

Then I remembered that I didn't know how to do any of those things. I wasn't Nike, and I didn't have a million-dollar marketing budget. The discrepancy between what I *thought* the video would look like and what it would *actually* look like would be the difference between a Michael Phelps Super Bowl ad and a finalist for *America's Funniest Home Videos*. I had to go back to the drawing board.

Then I heard a voice in my head tell me, "Make it funny. Wear a Speedo."

That's right. I heard the voice of God, and He told me to wear a Speedo. Well, technically, I think He was encouraging me to be genuine, but maybe God knows that I'm slow to understand so He has to be ridiculously specific sometimes.

Instead of doing what every other hopeful would try to do—present themselves as serious people doing important things—I took the contrarian approach and demonstrated that a triathlon is an inherently silly thing. We dress in Lycra and do three consecutive sports for ten or more hours, punishing ourselves in the name of extreme fitness. That's silly. Triathletes are silly people doing a silly thing, and we must not take ourselves too seriously. That was my approach, and it would serve as a contrast to my very serious history of alcohol abuse and anxiety.

The audition video, which lives on in perpetuity through the glory of YouTube (titled "Quest for Kona - Adam Hill" for anyone who cares to look for it), begins on a serious note as I talk about how Ironman has been a great supplement to sobriety. I slowly mount the treadmill and the bike trainer as "The Blue Danube" by Johann Strauss II begins to play in the background. Then comes a montage of me in a Speedo as I continue to narrate how my life of sobriety has led to further transformation. I sweep the floors in a Speedo, shave my legs in a Speedo, answer phone calls in a Speedo, eat dinner (a plate of bananas) in a Speedo, and journal in a Speedo. Then, for the purposes of establishing credibility, I do some "gratuitous bragging" by detailing my progression in the sport to demonstrate that I am right on the bubble of qualifying for Kona. Finally, I wrap it up by outlining my lofty goals for the season: win my age group, finish a race in under nine hours, and, of course, qualify for Kona.

I sent the video on to the casting agents with a hopeful attitude but low expectations. Honestly, I couldn't picture NBC or the Ironman people actually considering me based on this video. I had fun making it, and that would probably be the end of it.

Unexpectedly, however, I received an email from a man by the name of Eban Hathaway, a producer for the *Ironman: Quest for Kona* project. I was simultaneously brimming with excitement and scared shitless.

He informed me over the email that I was in the top twenty for consideration. He wanted to schedule a Skype call with my family and me to get a good feel for who we were.

Yikes.

As a family, we're fine on scripted videos, but in real time? We could be a bit unpredictable.

Now, it's worth pointing out that when I saw the second season of *The Real World* on MTV, I secretly wanted to be on that show. Granted, I was twelve years old when the show came out, and the desire left me once reality television evolved into mindless garbage that consisted of mindless people doing mindless things. I got older, and the show lost all depth and meaning and simply became a vessel for debauchery and douchey shenanigans.

Quest for Kona reignited that desire in me, and it offered a way for me to share my story and hopefully help others understand that there was a glorious alternative to fear and substance abuse. To make the cut, however, I had to impress Mr. Hathaway and the people at Ironman and NBC.

Eban couldn't have been more charming and professional. He was one of the producers responsible for the famed NBC broadcast of the Ironman World Championship, the same broadcast that beckoned me to the sport. How surreal it was that I was being interviewed by the producer of the very show that featured the amazing people that ignited a flame in my heart to chase the Kona dream? Here I was auditioning to be on a show that he was producing. I was starstruck, and it probably showed in the interview.

Regardless of how nerdy I may have come off and how abnormally quiet my kids were, the interview seemed to go very well. We would now have to wait another week before learning our fate. Either we would make the show and begin filming the training process, or I wouldn't, and it would be like the whole process never happened.

The next week I received a call from Eban, and I eagerly answered. I risked the question: "What's the word?"

"Well, I can't say yet," Eban said. "But we need to get you on a Skype call for another interview tomorrow."

Oh no, I thought, *another interview.*

That could only mean that they were on the fence about me and had to look for something that was missing from the first interview. What was it? Was I not charming enough? Did I not have the TV face? Did I say "um" too many times? Worse still, I would have to play the waiting game for a longer period of time while the bigwigs decided my fate.

"No problem," I lied as we concluded the call. I would be sweating bullets for another night.

The next day, I took a deep breath, opened my Skype account, and awaited the call. The goofy little chime sounded, and an icon appeared on my desktop, and I answered the call apprehensively. A woman with a South African accent was the first to speak.

"Hello, Adam! This is Paula Newby-Fraser."

"What the?" I muttered.

I was shaken out of my seat for a moment. *Did she just say what I thought she said? This definitely isn't Eban, and I think she said her name was Paula Newby-Fraser. As in, eight-time*

Ironman World Champion and arguably the most recognizable
person in the triathlon community.

"Hello, Adam? Are you there?" I was brought back to life as the voice on the other end of the line politely tried to get my attention.

"Uh...yeah! Sorry...I, uh, wasn't expecting...Well, how are you?" I fumbled with the video button, trying to figure out why I couldn't see Mrs. Newby-Fraser on my Skype screen. Meanwhile, she could see me and probably misinterpreted my look of confusion as disgust, or perhaps indigestion, but she proceeded despite the strange look on my face.

I was shocked for a number of reasons. First, I was expecting another interview, so I had on my guarded-yet-energetic face, awaiting the hardball questions about my alcoholism and triathlon career. Mostly, though, I was shocked because Paula Newby-Fraser was talking to me. I watched replays of her Kona wins incessantly during my build up to my first Ironman.

"Adam, I'm pleased to inform you that you have been selected as a cast member for *Ironman: Quest for Kona*," she told me.

The rest was a bit of a blur. I'm sure there was additional small talk and congratulations. I know she said that she would shake my hand if I made it to Kona. She may have even commented on my audition video.

Oh my God, I thought to myself. *Paula Newby-Fraser saw a video of me in a Speedo.*

It was about to get even more bizarre. I was going to be the first cast member "revealed" to the world through Ironman's website and social media. After my story was briefly introduced on Facebook, Instagram, and the Ironman website, I received messages of support and encouragement from people I didn't know. It was my first, albeit minor, experience as a small-scale celebrity, and it was fun.

I learned over the course of the next couple weeks the identities of my fellow castmates: a mother of a special needs child and autism ninja, a combat veteran helping soldiers with PTSD, a paraplegic handcycle athlete, an Australian model and actress, a Brazilian father and triathlete, a grandfather who became fit in his fifties, a mother who overcame postpartum depression through fitness, a triathlon coach from Malaysia, and a South American talk show host and celebrity.

All I knew at the time was that I didn't feel worthy to be chosen among these amazing people. What I didn't know was that these people would become my tribe.

I felt a strong desire to reach out to all of them and congratulate them as they were announced. Eric Beach, the combat veteran from Wisconsin, suggested we start a private Facebook group so that all of the cast members could share their experiences and we could be there to support one another. I was all in since I didn't know what to expect from this show. This was, by far, one of the best decisions we could have made together.

Meanwhile, I was critically thinking about my next steps as a triathlon coach and how I wanted to add value to the saturated coaching market. Within the broad spectrum of fitness coaching, I saw a lot of dangerous trends, some of which I fell for in my not-so-healthy days. For one, most fitness programs focused on the "no pain, no gain" approach to fitness. The idea that punishing oneself and performing with maximum effort or doing dangerous moves just because they look cool was the norm. I saw a way in which Extra Life Fitness could be different while making a difference.

If I could take the philosophies that changed my paradigm of fitness and apply it to my coaching, I knew lives could be changed. If people were really going to make sustainable transformations, they had to build a solid foundation, not punish themselves with dangerous routines that lead to injury or burnout in "ninety days or less." Nor would overly complicated diets that skirted around the primary issues be a sustainable solution. Aerobic fitness, simple nutrition, and mindfulness were the answer to sustainable lifestyle changes. That would be the approach of Extra Life Fitness.

It was a bold action and an audacious goal. I was launching out in faith: faith in myself and my ability to defy the odds. I believed that aerobic triathlon fitness could become a mainstream lifestyle, not just a niche hobby. I believed that triathletes were the fittest people in the world. Most importantly, I believed that anybody could participate. I had big plans for Extra Life Fitness.

My next step, now that I had a platform with *Quest for Kona*, was to develop undeniable credibility. Qualifying for Kona would cement my credibility and demonstrate that if it is possible for a hopeless alcoholic like myself, it is possible for anyone. Qualifying for Kona no longer felt like a dream; it became part of a mission. I was going to qualify for Kona, and I was going to do it on national fucking television.

Now all I needed was a race. I thought about racing at Ironman Coeur d'Alene, the iconic race in a beautiful region of Idaho, but for scheduling purposes (and as an effort to promote a new race in the Ironman circuit), I was offered a spot to race at Ironman Santa Rosa.

Santa Rosa would be a great option for me. I raced in the same region at Vineman the year before and finished in sixth place. This gave me a hefty dose of confidence.

Over the previous two years of training, I worked hard to try to find that 10 percent improvement that would put me into the Kona hunt and I was gaining ground. I proceeded to put together a rigorous training program for myself to maximize my potential. More important than the physical training was the mental priming I imposed on myself. I tried to block all limiting beliefs and replace them with empowering beliefs. This included believing that I could win the race outright. That was my goal. Win the freaking race. Shoot for the stars, and I may just make it to the moon.

It would help that the whole process was being filmed. This wasn't just another milestone I wanted to conquer on my own. This was going to be televised. I was going to be filmed from the start of my training to the finish line of the race, and that offered me a new level of accountability that I didn't previously have. I couldn't afford not to give it everything I had.

The project was a combination of self-shot footage during training and daily life, mixed in with interviews and race footage.

For a few months of 2017, I was the guy shamelessly taking self-ies while posing in my Speedo, riding my bike, or running with the beach in the background. Despite my best efforts, it was hard to avoid the critical stares of onlookers as I tried my best to channel my inner social media "influencer."

I did have a little bit of practice with filming myself previously, mainly for stupid videos I posted on triathlon pages just to be funny. Most were parodies or self-deprecating videos highlighting the general silliness of triathlon as a sport. Now it was different. I had to take it seriously...kinda.

Filming myself actually made training pretty interesting and productive. With the camera on, I was hyper-focused on good form. I also wasn't afraid to ham it up a bit for the camera to make it a little more entertaining. Let's face it, the excitement of watching a person ride their bike or run on a treadmill wanes pretty quickly. Fortunately, I didn't have to do all the filming on my own. Eban came to San Clemente for a few days to get the professional shots.

This was exciting. It was one thing to be filming myself, but now I had a guy with a camera follow me around in a totally non-creepy way.

Eban arranged his visit around my workout and life sched-ule to make the most out of his and my training time. Our first meeting happened at our local pool where he filmed me doing laps. As with most of my successful introductions during periods of Ironman training, I met Eban in person for the first time while wearing a Speedo. As he started unloading his gear, the reality of my situation hit me. I was going to be on a TV show. The excitement was overwhelming to say the least.

"Now, a few ground rules," Eban said to me. "First rule is this: try not to look at the camera. I know that sounds like an easy rule to follow, but inevitably every single time I do this, the person I'm filming catches the camera in the corner of their eye, and they look straight at it. It kills the shot. It's like a magnet."

"Okay, no problem," I said. I mean, how hard could it really be to avoid looking at the camera?

"Second rule: just be yourself. Don't try to look more badass than you already are because it will show on camera. The camera doesn't just add fifteen pounds; it magnifies everything."

Noted. Don't be a douche. Check.

With those ground rules established, I jumped into the water and started swimming as naturally as I could, a task made all the more difficult by the fact that my every move was being documented by an expensive, high-resolution camera. I didn't see it, but I knew it was there, and it made me extremely self-conscious.

I then became aware of a small rectangular box about two inches from my forehead, moving along at the same pace as my rate of swim speed. It did not interfere with my stroke, but I kept wanting to adjust my stroke to avoid hitting it. My efforts were unnecessary though because Eban was all over it like the pro he was.

Then I came to the wall and stopped for a rest. So, too, did the camera, still within two inches of my face. It was right there in my periphery.

Don't look at it. Don't look at it, I repeated to myself. Then I looked right at it.

"Shit!" I muttered.

"Every single time!" Eban laughed.

That was the last time I looked at the camera. I suppose subconsciously I just had to get it out of my system.

For the remainder of the week, I was filmed swimming, biking, running, doing strength training, eating eggs, walking with my family, pretending to eat ice cream (okay, *actually* eating ice cream), and working with athletes I coached. The whole time I was able to master the "workout intensity" face and avoid looking at the camera. In the process, I had a week of really, really well-focused training. Few things work better to help me focus on form and quality than a man filming my every move during a workout.

I have immense gratitude for Eban Hathaway. While I've never been in the film industry, I've heard stories of reality TV producers who lack empathy or compassion for their subjects. Eban couldn't have been more different from that stereotype. He believed in me and my fellow castmates. He fought for us, led us when we needed to be led, and gave us room when we needed space. Most of all, he understood and had a passion for the subject he was producing. It was clear by his actions. The support that he gave me had a clear impact on my ability to train just a little harder to attain that 10 percent I needed to be in the hunt for an Ironman win and a ticket to Kona.

It is never enough just to set an ambiguous goal to be faster, better, or stronger. The question is "Why?" Why is it necessary?

That why has to be compelling—compelling enough to get my ass out of bed when I would rather sleep in. Compelling enough to force me to push on even when it gets challenging—and it will get challenging. When the body and mind say, "*Quit! Quit! Quit,*" the compelling reason behind my why lights the fire in my heart that pushes me forward. It's the compelling why that gets 300 watts of power out of me when my brain tells me that 290 is too much.

Without a compelling why, we lose the game before we even get started.

My why was compelling enough for me to push through the most intense pain brought on by Ironman training so that that physical pain was barely uncomfortable at all. I knew what real pain was. I associated so much pain with the person I used to be and so much joy with the person I was becoming. I wanted to sprint toward that person as fast as I possibly could, regardless of the obstacles. I wanted to be the example that taught my kids that overcoming challenges is a beautiful and fulfilling part of life and they can do anything they feel a passion and a drive for. I wanted to continue imprinting these healthy habits so I could fortify my sobriety. Thankfully, it was working.

To top it off, I wanted to prove to others what is possible beyond fear and addiction.

Now I had a platform. I had an audience of people who might be struggling with addiction, anxiety, or depression who would hear my story and watch as I attempted to achieve a challenging goal. That would hold me accountable to my goal. Accountability is hugely important. There have to be real consequences for not achieving a goal and real rewards for achieving it. Mine were very public, and my coaching credibility was at stake.

In addition to having a compelling why, I needed the goal to be specific. My goal, which I stated as frequently as I could as if achieving it were a given, was to finish Ironman Santa Rosa in nine hours. That would be a one-hour swim, a 4:40 bike, and a 3:15 run (plus some extra time for transitions). I taped these times to the front of my bike trainer so that I could always see them. I trained as if I was already a nine-hour Ironman. While I don't recommend this exact approach for athletes I coach (I do recommend the visualization, but the method I outline here increases the likelihood of injury or burnout, so extreme attention has to be given to recovery, diet, and overall health), I made my interval and threshold sessions much harder to reach my targets. Instead of running on the road or track for interval sessions, I used a treadmill so I could force faster paces. My threshold sessions were now done at a 6:20 minute per mile pace. Additionally, I increased my FTP from 275 to 300 watts over the course of the training build.

The swim was still a big question mark. I made dramatic improvements in my first years as a triathlete, to the point where I was swam sub-1:10 Ironman swim splits. For some reason, however, I plateaued and regressed a little bit. Anxiety crept back into my open-water swims, and panic attacks started to occur more frequently. During a half Ironman in St. George, Utah, I panicked early in the swim and had to grab a kayak.

Visions of the 2012 Ironman in that same venue came flooding through my mind. I saw videos of that year's race many times. The start of the race was as calm as could be. Swimmers ventured out into their 2.4-mile swim with crystal clear, flat waters. Halfway through, the wind picked up, and Sand Hollow Reservoir turned into a washing machine of swells and chop. Swimmers had to be rescued left and right, and visibility became an issue.

I read horror stories from some of the racers, some of which were probably embellished, but seemed all too real as I sat bobbing up and down in that very same body of water. There was a light chop, and my brain told me that a severe windstorm was inevitable, and I would be left flailing about, forgotten by the race officials, in the middle of the lake until a terrifying doom overcame me, and I would sink into the murky depths.

I held onto that kayak for dear life until I collected myself. Then I went off again and swam for a bit until the panic once again took me, at which point I grabbed another kayak. So went the remainder of that agonizing swim.

Unfortunately, that experience seemed to imprint the fear of swimming back into me, and the timing could not have been worse. I was a mere two months from my qualifying race in Santa Rosa.

Anxiety is a strange thing. Our brains tell us to worry about the dumbest things rather than focusing on the things that should actually worry us. Swimming in a race is relatively safe. There is support everywhere and very little chance that anything bad will happen. Yet my anxiety decided to anchor to the swim. I worried about the overwhelming reality that I was trying to start a successful fitness coaching business and the fact that I was about to reveal my entire self to the world through *Quest for Kona*. If I failed, it would be televised. The fact that I was floating in the middle of the water without any support, except from my own abilities, was perhaps analogous to the fact that I could trust only myself and my abilities. I was confident in myself and my ability to succeed on my own, but the fear just seemed to manifest itself in the water. Naturally, my swim speed suffered.

Still, I was right on the bubble. Even if my swim were slower, I had the bike power and run capabilities to achieve my goals and take home a KQ, a Kona Qualification...*if* I executed the race perfectly.

After months of training, filming, and preparing, the qualifying race in Santa Rosa was nearly upon me. The schedule was set. Eban and his team of producers had cleared all of the details of the filming with Ironman. I had done everything I could possibly do. Now all I had to do was breathe. I was ready, as long as I could overcome my mind.

Running Strong

IRONMAN ARIZONA, 2016. MILE 114.

Exiting Transition 2 (T2), I did my ritual system check: no stomach issues, no cramping, breathing rate normal, and plenty of energy. Everything was feeling good after the bike ride as I began the long 26.2-mile run on a perfectly cool Tempe, Arizona, afternoon.

This system check was pivotal. It was one of the determining factors of whether this was going to be a great day or a really bad day.

During my previous five system checks at full Ironman races, there were two races where I immediately felt terrible and proceeded to have the longest, most painful runs of my life. It was these experiences that I wanted to avoid. Even though I survived the remaining three marathons, I never felt like I fully reached my potential on the run.

In this particular race, coming out of T2, I felt better than ever at the beginning of a run. Even though I felt great, I backed off the pace (or so I thought) during the first mile. While the Ironman Arizona run is advertised as flat, the first couple miles have a few small bumps, which serve to break up the pace a bit.

I was surprised to see as I ran past the first mile that I did so at a 7:19 pace.

Shit, that's too fast.

I surprised myself. Usually, I was demoralized to see an Ironman pace well below my training paces, but today I had far exceeded any pace logged in my long run training. It scared me a little. I backed off the pace a bit more. While I felt good, I didn't want to inadvertently blow myself up early in the run, only to walk the remainder of the marathon.

I ran through mile two at a pace of 7:17.

Well, that didn't work. Let's try backing off the pace a little more.

Mile 3, 7:15.

Okay, this was ridiculous. At that point, I was resigned to the fact that I would just be running these super awesome paces during the course of the race. It was clear that the first couple miles were not an anomaly, and I was truly running well. But with the paranoia of an anticipated bonk later in the race, I found myself fearful that I was self-sabotaging.

I ran with careful confidence for the first half of the run until I was sure I could sustain the pace. I wasn't being punked by my body or swindled by my fitness. *I was really doing it. I was running well off the bike in an Ironman!*

At Mile 13.1, I decided to kick it up a notch. In an effort not to slow down, I increased my rate of breathing to two steps for every breath in and out. This set me up for a good rhythm to continue running my sub-7:30 pace.

I took that moment to internalize how it felt to run well off the bike and maintain a good rhythm. I now had a point of reference, and I wanted to imprint it in my psyche for all of my future Ironman marathons. If I could continue to repeat this success in future races, the Kona dream would be mine.

13

THE RACE
OF MY LIFE

"I can't do this," I cried into the arms of my wife as we sat in the parking lot of Lake Sonoma on the morning of July 29, 2017, the day of Ironman Santa Rosa.

I was melting down, and the race hadn't even started yet. The pressure was all piling up. I knew that a cameraman was waiting for me in transition, readying himself to film every single thing I did on this day; good and bad, ups and downs, success or failure. It was hitting me hard in a brief moment of self-pity and debilitating fear.

I was in the best physical shape of my life. From a training perspective, I uncovered the 10 percent I needed, nestled away in minor improvements. A person doesn't find the final 10 percent through some huge revelation. Usually, it's through a number of small tweaks that compound into huge results. I was stronger on the bike than I'd ever been before. I'd never been faster on the run. My nutrition was nailed down. I was set to achieve all my goals, except for one. The swim.

The swim still eluded me. I discovered the secret of a fast swim time once before, swimming a 1:03 at Vineman a year earlier. Then in one season, it was gone, having evaporated with my confidence. I knew that a poor swim time could break my chances at a KQ. I talked a big game of breaking nine hours, but if I came out of the water any slower than 1:10, I wouldn't even be in the running for Kona, let alone a nine-hour Ironman finish. The whole race was riding on my ability to get my ass around the swim course in under an hour and ten minutes.

I finished my meltdown and quietly made the walk down to the transition area. During the walk, I told myself that I could have my freak out, but that would be the only one for the day. Once I crossed into transition, it was game on. Absolute focus. Confidence. Power.

Take. No. Prisoners.

It was a controlled moment of weakness, and then I made a decision not to be afraid anymore. Just like when I had made the decision to stop drinking, the decision not to fear was entirely in my control. Even if the conditions of the race were not in my control, I would not be a slave to my brain. I was living a life with intention. I had a purpose for today, and I was going to make every second of it count.

Walking down the hill, I felt timid, anxious, and nervous. I crossed into transition and put on my game face. My focus shifted to the minute details in front of me at that very moment. Get to my bike. Check the components. Fill my water bottles. Get my swim gear ready. Use the toilet. Use the toilet again.

Okay, maybe use the toilet one more time.

Eban followed me around for a bit with the camera while I prepared myself in transition, but thankfully he allowed me to use the toilet in peace. It's a sacred tradition every triathlete must follow. It's the pre-race "release" of nervous energy within the darkened confines of the porta potty. There is no room for germaphobia in a triathlon, especially during the pre-race constitution. In the days leading up to a race, I do everything to protect myself from germs short of armoring myself in bubble wrap. On race day, however, the most unsanitary of toilet seats are fair game.

Transition was surprisingly a little less hectic with the camera on me than previous races. I just wasn't conscious of it. I was obsessively focused. Obsessive focus is my superpower, and I was in my zone. It was comforting to have Eban there. He had been something of a training partner for those last few months, someone I always checked in with. Someone who encouraged and supported me.

I left transition as the light of the morning peeked into existence and displayed the outline of the Lake Sonoma hilltops. It was a long and steep quarter mile walk down the boat ramp to the swim entry area, an ominous walk that foreshadowed the inevitable slog back up the ramp, which would take place after swimming 2.4 miles.

Down at the swim start, I donned my sleeveless wetsuit. The water was a toasty seventy-six degrees, just slightly below the wetsuit legal limit. The morning air temperature was just over fifty degrees, but the sun would come up later, and the temperature would shoot up to well over eighty. Even with the crispness of the morning air, the seventy-six-degree water would host a very warm swim. Sleeveless was the way to go.

The weather was calm and clear before the race started as athletes trickled down the boat ramp to the swim corral. The corral, as it is lovingly called, is the area where athletes queue up to start their day. The line of athletes extended a few hundred yards, all ordered by projected swim time. If an athlete thought they would finish the swim in under an hour, they would line up in the "less than sixty minutes" section. If they planned to finish in a time of 1:05, they would line up in the "1:00–1:10" section. Over the course of a half hour, the race officials slowly let the athletes trickle into the water to start, thus spreading out the field of athletes. I chose to line up at the very front of the 1:00–1:10 section.

The sub-one-hour swimmers were primarily "fish," or lifelong swimmers, and had skills that I had yet to master, so lining up with them would have been optimistic to say the least. Yet the 1:00–1:10 group was right where I had been swimming when I swam well. Lining up at the very front of the group provided me a couple advantages. First, I would get a draft effect from the slightly faster swimmers getting out ahead of me (I would rather be swum over than have to swim over people). More importantly, I would have a greater chance of catching up with the lead cyclists early. I've been in too many situations where I had a slow swim time and then had to spend half of the bike ride passing people, exerting vast amounts of energy. Not this time. Instead, I took as much of an advantage as I could from the rolling swim start, keeping the majority of the athletes behind me. Even if I was passed, I could very quickly catch up on the bike.

There's a quiet solitude that exists at the starting line of a race. Maybe it's the earplugs that muffle the nervous energy. Maybe it's the adrenaline masking the rapid beating of the heart. Maybe it is the brief pause of the techno music while the color guard is readied for "The Star-Spangled Banner." Regardless, it's a moment of peace that represents absolute surrender to the fact that there's no turning back. All the worrying about the things that are out of our human control—the weather, the temperature of the water, the wind, mechanical issues, sickness, and everything else—is all in the past, and only acceptance of the present reality exists. The work has been done, the stage is set, and God has put forth His profound grace on this day and allowed us the strength to do this beautiful, crazy, magical, empowering thing. The only option is to move forward in faith and confidence.

I stood nestled together in an orgy of neoprene. At the start, we're all alone. Anonymous. Strangers in the same black wetsuits and the same pink or green swim caps. We beat each other up as strangers in the swim, slowly come to know each other on the bike as our identities emerged, develop camaraderie on the run, and then finally become family in victory at the finish line. It's a beautiful thing, and it's analogous to the human experience we all have as we evolve through our personal stories.

Though I had my support team, my family, and the crew of *Quest for Kona* behind me, I was all alone in that moment, and it's exactly where I wanted and needed to be.

Then came the blast of the cannon.

For most of the age groupers, save for the ten to fifteen people right at the front of the corral, the cannon firing doesn't really mean anything at the immediate moment. It's not like we all jump in the water at once. It's only a signal that the line is going to start moving at some point in the near future. For a few more minutes, I continued to stand there as I saw a line of white water begin to form at the entrance of the lake and extend outward into an arrow. Then we shuffled forward ever so slowly, passive-aggressively fighting for a slightly better position in the line leading up to the start of the race. I weighed my options for whom I would like to have kick me in the face as I maneuvered myself behind certain individuals.

Before too long, I was under the arch and a volunteer shouted, "Go, go, go!" as I dove in and began taking my first few strokes, awkwardly trying to avoid being hit by a stray foot or hand. No matter how much training or preparation takes place beforehand, the first few hundred yards of the swim will invariably consist of the brain ping-ponging between *I'm drowning, I've got this, I can't breathe, What the fuck am I doing?*, and *What if there's a tidal wave that hits us during this lake swim?* That's just the reality of it, and I have to deal with it. The key is to never allow myself to negotiate with my brain. As silly as it sounds, we can't let our brains win because the brain will always seek the path of least resistance. In this case, that would be quitting and jumping onto a kayak. Repeat after me: when shit gets hard, say, "Fuck off, brain. I've got this."

I just had to shut it off and keep going. Decide to push through it. Have faith that the fear will pass, and trust in the training. One stroke at a time. That's what I did.

Around the first turn buoy, about four hundred meters from shore, I finally started to get into a comfortable rhythm. I taught myself to practice a higher turnover in open-water swims to maintain momentum and increase the frequency of breaths. Oddly, the faster, less powerful swim stroke seemed more comfortable. It was like a faster cadence on the run at a slower speed. Over time, it developed into greater comfort and increased paces.

I swam comfortably and at a high tempo, but I was still passed frequently. It was a frustrating reality for me but one I accepted as normal. After all, I started toward the front of the pack for this very reason. I would catch them on the bike.

As we made a right turn after the first turn buoy, it was a long swim to the next turn, about eight hundred meters. Then it was a right turn for about a couple hundred meters and a final turn toward the start/finish, where we began our second loop. It was during this leg back to the start where it got challenging.

The sun was now up over the mountains, and the warmth of the water, combined with the coolness of the air, caused a thick and bright haze to form over the water. Every time we looked up to get a sight line, we were met with bright white haze and silhouetted figures flailing about. I had to depend on my neighbors and the occasional marker buoy to make sure that I was on the right track.

Back at the swim finish, I and my neoprene-clad siblings exited the water briefly to run over a timing mat, only to get back in the water and swim the same course again. Multiple-loop swim courses are always a special challenge because they add an extra element of demoralization. Briefly exiting the water is a tremendous mindfuck, one that breaks a swimmer's rhythm. It's a ceremonious, "You're halfway done, jerk! Now get back out there and suffer some more!" To add insult to injury, in races with a rolling start, where the slowest swimmers are entering the water twenty to thirty minutes behind the fastest swimmers, it is inevitable that the faster swimmers will run into a brick wall of slower swimmers just starting their race. It's as if the final 250 miles of the Daytona 500 were raced in Los Angeles rush-hour traffic.

About a third of the way into my second loop, I ran into my first set of slower swimmers. It was hard to avoid, and I felt really terrible about it because most of those swimmers were battling their own anxieties on the swim only to have an armada of fish plow through them. In my defense, it was impossible to know that I was coming up on another swimmer when my eyes were down and the water was a mixture of bubbles and murkiness. The only solution was to essentially swim over people. I stopped a few times to reroute myself because the number of people in front of me was just so thick. I exerted a lot more energy with little or no benefit as I swam sideways, backtracked, and generally fought my way forward.

This time, the glare from the haze was much worse, and the frantic splashing from more and more athletes did not help things. It was nearly impossible to tell which direction was right with everyone swimming in so many different directions. Finally, I rounded the last buoy and headed toward the swim exit and boat ramp. The last few hundred yards of the swim toward the exit always felt like the longest stretch of the swim. At that point, I just did my best to will myself forward despite tired arms. I eased up my stroke and started kicking to get the blood to my legs to help ease the shock of jumping from a horizontal to a vertical position and starting to run.

My fingertips grazed the serrated concrete floor of the boat ramp that rapidly sloped upward toward the exit. This was my cue to stand up and start running. With two or three awkward hops to clear my feet from the water, I started to run. I glanced quickly at my time.

1:10.

It was right at the slow end of where I needed to finish. I was hoping for 1:05 or faster, and 1:10 was the slowest I could swim and still have a slim shot of catching the leaders. I would have my work cut out for me on the bike.

In reality, the time on the clock doesn't hold too much meaning. There are a lot of factors that can affect a swim time one way or another. The course may have been longer; the conditions could be an issue; the water could have a consistency similar to maple syrup. Well, some issues are more likely than others, but there are factors that could have affected everyone's swim time...Or it could have been just me. There was no way to know until I could infer a conclusion later in the race.

There's no point in dwelling on it, I thought to myself. *It was a slow swim. Deal with it and move on. Crush the bike and hold on for the run.*

After running up the quarter-mile boat ramp to the transition area, my heart rate was the highest it would ever be in the race. That was okay. It was normal. The key was to let it drop down on the bike as I descended into the valley. For now, I just needed to get to my bike.

I ran into transition and was met by the cameraman, Trent, who was chasing me while dodging bikes in and out of T1, all the way to the changing tent where we briefly left each other. Unlike my first experiences with transition areas, the changing process had become automatic for me: unload the bag, put on helmet, apply some Vaseline to junk, grab bike shoes, and go. My bike was fairly close to the bike exit so it would be easier to run while carrying my shoes and then put them on when I got to my bike. Running while wearing bike shoes is a cute and funny little adventure that cyclists can relate to. It somewhat resembles an oddly clad Fred Astaire rushing off stage to use the bathroom after holding it for an entire show. Holding my bike shoes, I ran a lot faster with a lot less awkwardness.

I got out of the changing tent and ran to my bike. Trent was waiting for me at my bike setup. We wouldn't be there long. I put on my shoes, grabbed my bike, and left the transition area. During the whole run to the bike mount, Trent followed alongside me in extreme close-up mode, and I kept thinking to myself, *please don't trip...Please don't trip...*

Successful with the not-tripping endeavor, I mounted my bike at the appropriate time and started grinding around the short turns to the bike course. After the first couple turns out of transition, passing a few people on the way out, I made it to the bridge that I just swam under.

As I looked over the bridge at the lake I just exited, the enormity of the race struck me. I saw the tiny forms of hundreds of humans still swimming, still challenging themselves, still overcoming fear, covering a vast distance. It was a sobering moment as I realized that some of them would be in the water for more than two hours. Some would be on the entire course for seventeen hours. There I was complaining about my 1:10 swim. Man, was I lucky to be there.

It's funny to think through what we tend to complain about and how it is shaped by our perspective. I was racing in this Ironman Triathlon, something that 99.999 percent of the world will never do, challenging the leaders, something even fewer people will ever do, and my first thought went to what I *wasn't* able to accomplish. The practice of gaining perspective is important in all areas of life, lest we risk a constant sense of demoralization. We are constantly looking up at what we haven't yet achieved or received and associating a sense of loss with that thing. Rarely do people actually stop to look back on what they have gained. This shift in perspective starts with gratitude. We have to battle back the constant misinformation coming from our brains telling us that we're not good enough and begin with the appreciation of all that we have received or accomplished. For me, I was damn grateful to be racing an Ironman and chasing down the leaders of the race, something that would not have been possible if I hadn't got sober and began believing in myself.

Trent and his motorcycle escort pulled up on me just then and snapped me out of my momentary reflection and back to the task at hand. He was sitting backward on a motorcycle being driven by a former highway patrol officer. I imagine that over the course of a five-hour Ironman bike leg, as he looked through the viewfinder of a camera for nearly that whole time, he was trying desperately not to puke. The motorcycle escort also had a very careful job to do. First, he could not interfere with any athletes. This meant he had to carefully navigate around and between athletes as they passed each other and tried to run their own race. Second, he couldn't ride in front of me because it would give me a draft advantage. He had to stay either at my side or behind me.

Third, and probably most difficult, he had to anticipate my moves. He did all of these things flawlessly.

I was insanely focused during this portion of the race. What else could I do? I had a freaking camera in my face for most of the ride. Five hours on a bike is a long time, and one can do a lot of crazy shit when out on the road all alone. Sometimes I sing to myself, make conversation with people in my head, and dance a little. With my ego fully attentive to the fact that people would watch this, I had to avoid the temptation to do something silly. In retrospect, I probably would have made the show more entertaining if I injected a little more reality into it.

Instead, I stared straight ahead, donning my "intense racer" face. I was a man on a mission, passing cyclists constantly, which made me look like a rocket ship. Coming off a lackluster swim, darting through the field of racers on the bike was great for television and my confidence.

There was really no way for me to know how well I was doing on the bike leg. I felt good. Nutrition was going down fine and not coming back up. My heart rate was on track, and I was passing riders, but as an amateur among two thousand athletes, it was impossible to know my place on the bike leg unless I came out of the water at the very front, which did not happen.

The rolling start doesn't help matters. Technically, someone could start the race after me and beat me even though they finished after me. The best I could do was just race my race, and not focus on anybody else...and keep my eyes off the freaking camera.

The first half of the Ironman Santa Rosa bike course was rolling through the beautiful hillsides and vineyards of Sonoma. It was poetic, really. When I was a drinker, I was partial to wine.

For some reason, I had fewer "incidents" with wine. Hard alcohol got me drunk too quickly, and the anxiety attacks I experienced after a night of drinking it were far more severe. With beer, I lost all bladder control. I had to urinate every fifteen minutes, and when I passed out, I inevitably wet the bed. Those effects happened less often when I drank wine. Plus, it had the added benefit (at least from my screwed-up perception) that I was a connoisseur of the finer things and therefore "in control." At the grocery store, I held a bottle of wine, reading the description, which made me look distinguished. In reality, I was checking the alcohol content. Many bottles advertise 13.5 percent alcohol while some had upwards of 15 percent. Always a value shopper, I looked for the latter. Yes, I am a real alcoholic.

I wondered for a moment where I would be if I were still drinking. I sure as hell wouldn't be doing this race. *Would I be in jail? Would I be dead?*

I pictured myself lying passed out in one of the gutters on the side of the road next to a vineyard. The beautiful trees, hillsides, and peaceful surroundings would mask the pain, suffering, and chaos going on within me. All these Ironman athletes would pass by my inebriated corpse, looking on with pity at the wasted life. I, too, pitied what could have been. By grace, it wasn't, and I was allowed to leave those vineyards behind me, both literally and figuratively.

Finishing the first half of the course, we headed back into Santa Rosa for two loops around town. At that moment, a problem began to present itself. I was out of nutrition. I had prepared two bottles, one that I would have for the first half of the bike race, and the second that I would pick up from the special needs station.

A special needs station is an aid station that can be accessed about halfway through the race. It is where a racer can store additional nutrition, extra bike parts, letters from family, or other things they might need for the remainder of the race. Most often they are placed at about mile 56.

At least I *thought* it was at mile 56.

At every other race I'd ever done, the bike special needs station was placed at about the halfway point of the bike segment, which made perfect sense. I planned every race to down one bottle for the first half and then one for the second half. I was now past mile 56, and the bike special needs was nowhere to be found.

Then came mile 60...then mile 65...still no special needs.

I feared that I missed it and was preparing contingency plans. *Could I switch to the on-course nutrition from the aid stations? Would that be enough?* I thought my race was fucked. Then, like an oasis, the bright-orange special-needs bags came into view in the distance. I sighed with relief that I would get my nutrition down. It came at mile 70, nearly fifteen miles after I had expected it. That amounted to about forty minutes of no nutritional intake, which was highly suboptimal.

I took the bottle and took a big gulp and went on my way, hoping there would be no lasting effects from the nutrition deficiency. I seemed to be doing okay. I wasn't losing any power, and my heart rate was not drifting downward. Both would be signs of not having enough fuel in the tank. I still felt strong, but I was ready to get off the bike, which was normal at about eighty miles in, but the real test would come on the run. I wouldn't find out if the missed nutrition would affect me until I got off my bike and started running.

Eighty miles into a 112-mile bike segment may sound like it's close to the end, but in reality, thirty-two miles is still a long way to ride. That's almost an hour and a half of riding still to go. It's best not to put into your mind the idea that "I'm almost there." Saying that tells our brains a false story, and you are not focused on the present moment. When you give up on the present, your performance suffers. I never give myself an excuse to coast. Any time a spectator says, "You're almost there," I ignore them. I know they mean well, but it's not a good thing to say to someone who still has many more miles to ride or run and needs to focus on the immediate present. I would love it if they would instead yell, "I have French fries!" and actually mean it, but sadly that hasn't happened.

All of that said, my butt really fucking hurt, and I wanted off the bike.

The quality of the roads during the last half of the bike ride did not help my sore ass situation. The roads hadn't been repaved since the original missionaries came through Santa Rosa hundreds of years prior. At least it felt that way. To top it off, we had to do two loops of it. The beauty of the vineyards and the smooth roads faded into the past as all of the cyclists came to accept their new and bumpy reality.

I rounded the final loop and headed into the last few miles of the bike course. We weaved through downtown Santa Rosa as crowds of onlookers held signs and rang cowbells. I felt a renewed sense of nervousness as I prepared to go for a little 26.2-mile run. *Would I be able to run well off the bike?* I would find out shortly.

I rounded the last corner to the straightaway that led to T2, and as I did, I heard Mike Riley, the famous "voice" of Ironman, shouting out the names of racers coming in. I came in right behind another athlete, dismounted, and parted with my bicycle as if I never wanted to see it again...or if I did, it would be in Kona. The bike was no longer my focus. It was time to run.

I race with a mantra: "Swim through the fear, bike with your brain, and run with your heart." So far, I accomplished the first two. Even though I finished the bike leg in 4:52, about five to ten minutes off my goal, my running legs felt strong, which was vastly more important than a fast bike split. In an event like Ironman, it's much more preferable to sacrifice ten minutes on the bike to have fresh running legs. It could net as much as a half hour or more on the run.

My brain had done its job, keeping me in control on the bike, but it was time to turn my brain off. The mind is a powerful thing when the body is experiencing pain, and it will tell us at every opportunity to end the pain by quitting, slowing down, or just taking a quick break. But the heart and the spirit, if their force is stronger than the mind, can lead us beyond our limits. It was time to run with the heart.

Eban met me in the T2 changing tent and immediately did an extreme close-up on my feet as I slipped on my running shoes. I pretended not to notice he was there, as I was trained to do, and quickly trotted out of the changing tent ahead of the person I came into the tent with. One target down.

I still didn't know what position I was in. There was nobody around me aside from one or two other racers up ahead and behind me, but I had been in this position before and still finished way behind the winners. I could be fifth or fiftieth for all I knew. The thirty-five to thirty-nine male age group is one of the fastest in every race, and often the overall winner will come from this age group, so I had to stay mindful of that possibility, and push my limits.

At around mile 3, I caught up with a friend who also happened to be in my age group and ran with him for a bit. He said he believed we were in fifth in our age group. This raised my spirits. I had never been that high in a race before. My first mile was a quick 7:12 minute per mile pace. The second mile was 7:14. I was on track to crush my 3:15 marathon goal as long as I could avoid slowing down.

Ironman marathons are different than traditional marathons because the goals are different. In an open marathon, the goal is to run as fast as possible for 26.2 miles. The whole race is between two and a half and five hours, so one can afford to push the effort well into the anaerobic zone. The goal in an Ironman marathon is to delay the process of slowing down for as long as possible, *not* run as fast as possible. The Ironman is already well over half over, and fatigue has already set in. It's a different mindset, one that requires a sharp focus on the systems in play: nutrition, physical state, core temperature, and many other things.

I was met by my cameraman friend, Trent, again at about mile 2.5. He drove right in front of me and gave me tremendous motivation. I pictured myself as the Terminator running down a motorcycle and continued to keep focus and form.

I settled into a comfortably hard 7:20–7:30 pace for the next few miles, but sadly, I had to say goodbye to my friend with the camera, at least until the second lap. Now it was time to run alone for a few miles. Running alone was something I was used to. I do all my training alone purposely so I can get comfortable with myself in the long portions of Ironman when I am next to nobody. It is my meditation, and a chance to find peace with my usually active mind. Santa Rosa had many "dead" zones (areas where there are limited spectators), and during the first loop of the course, there weren't many other racers nearby. Keeping peace with myself was a key part of my strategy.

Finally heading back into town around mile 8 to start the second loop, I met with lots of spectators. I caught my parents right around the turnaround area, and they began shouting at me "Fourth! Fourth!" At least that's what I think I heard from them. Was this fourth overall or in my age group? What if I was close to *winning* the race? This gave me both confidence and dread at the same time. While I was certainly happy to be in the hunt, I had to defend that position against some very hungry athletes. Many times, the advantage goes to the chaser, not the chased. Now that I *knew* the information, I knew it was mine to lose. I had eighteen more miles to hold this pace, gain position, and hold everyone else off. On to lap two.

I still felt strong, and I was still passing people, but I didn't know if those people were on their first or second lap. Since I was on my second and some people were just starting the run, it was difficult to distinguish between who was just starting and who was on the same loop as me. The important thing was that I wasn't getting passed.

I met back up with my trusted cameraman on the motor-cycle and got back to correcting my form for the camera. This loop had an added obstacle of people jumping out in front of me to get some camera time. They thought it was the highlight camera until I nearly ran into them. At that time, they thought I was the race leader. I have to admit, that was pretty cool. I heard some murmurs of, "He must be winning." They didn't know that I had already won because I had transformed my life.

I wasn't slowing down, which was good. I was holding steady with a 7:30 minute per mile pace, but I was definitely starting to feel it. The rest of that second loop and most of the third were a blur to me. My brain filled with nothing but shoddy arithmetic as to when I would arrive at the finish line. I was a machine.

I don't remember feeling any pain, but I know that I was pushing beyond my red line. My heart rate for most of the run was nearly 160, which is about what it would be for an open marathon, not a marathon run after a swim and a bike. I was channeling something much more than glycogen. I was channeling everything I had in me, knowing that this was the race where I would achieve my dream, and the whole thing would be televised.

I swam through fear, biked with my brain, and now I was running with my heart.

This was the moment. Transcending fear and addiction, transforming my health and fitness, becoming an Ironman triathlete, chasing the Kona dream, and now *Quest for Kona*; all of it culminating at that very moment as I approached the final mile to the finish of my life.

The Finish

IRONMAN SANTA ROSA, 2017. MILE 140.

After 25.5 miles of running, I finally turned off the Santa Rosa river trail and onto the main streets leading to my seventh Ironman finish line. As I ran by crowds of people, I approached an iconic sign. It read: "Laps 2 & 3: left, Finish line: right."

I ran by this sign two other times and turned left. It was a dreadful feeling knowing that the finish line was right there, but there were still many more miles to run. Finally, I got to take the *right* turn. As I did, my eyes started to water. I simultaneously felt stronger and weaker than I ever had in my life.

The tears that flowed in that last mile were tears of joy for the victories I achieved that day. Tears for transcending the fears that had overtaken me in the past few months and years. Tears of gratitude for my wife, kids, and family who stood beside me through all my challenges. Tears for the amazing life God granted me through His grace and through sobriety. Tears for having accomplished another amazing feat, all in front of the camera for the world to see.

I miscalculated how long the finish would take after that final turn. I assumed it was right around the corner, but it wasn't. I had to weave through a labyrinth of side streets to get to the finish. Around every turn, large crowds greeted me with cheers and cowbells. The contrasting feelings one has in these races are amazing, and at this time, I was feeling both numb and full of energy. As I ran through this labyrinth, a strange thought entered my mind.

What if I'm winning?

I hadn't seen anyone in front of me since I made the turn at the sign directing athletes to the finish. No athlete ever passed me on the run. There was a chance, albeit a small one, that I could be leading the race.

It was then that I thought I heard Mike Riley announce, "He's on his way, folks! Just a third of a mile more to go, and he'll be here!"

Now, he could have been talking about a high-profile racer, or maybe he said "she," or maybe it was the pizza delivery guy he was talking about, but at that moment, I felt like he was talking about me. I was winning the race, and I was going to be breaking the tape in just one-third of a mile.

It was a crazy thought, I know, but delusions are common in the last few hundred meters of an Ironman.

＝ 𝔬𝔬 ⅄

I ran down the finisher chute on the way toward those glorious arches. I reached my hands out to high five the crowd. Just then, I caught a glimpse of what was waiting for me beyond the finish line. There stood Eban, the producer of *Quest for Kona*, with a camera; Trent, the cameraman; and in front of them, my daughter holding a medal.

I couldn't hold it together. As I crossed the finish line, crying like a child, I collapsed into the arms of my nine-year-old, and she did her best to hold me up. I finally descended to the ground in a heap of joy and residual adrenaline. I had a mediocre 1:10 swim, a respectable 4:52 bike, and a smoking fast 3:16 run. My total time was 9:29, my second race in a row breaking 9:30.

Just finishing these races inspires a ton of gratitude and joy. Putting together a *great* race is many levels above that and brings about feelings that I can't put into words. It's a feeling I want everyone in the world to experience. It's a reason why I coach.

I was lying on the ground, making the medical personnel and race officials nervous about my well-being. My wife knelt down and whispered in my ear a single word, and it affirmed that I had just achieved my dream.

"Third!"

I was third place in my age group. I was seventeenth overall out of nearly two thousand people. The moment she told me that, I knew that I just achieved what I had set out to accomplish four and a half years earlier while sitting in my bed recovering from shoulder surgery. At that time, I was so embarrassed by the idea because I was in such poor shape. I had no business doing a triathlon, let alone an Ironman. Yet I still told myself that I would become an Ironman. Not only that—I committed to myself that I would qualify for Kona.

On July 29, 2017, I did just that.

The Kona rolldown presentation was rather anticlimactic. After so many years of working so hard to achieve this goal, it was reduced to sitting on a grassy knoll as Mike Riley read names off a list. I stood in line for about thirty minutes, waiting to part with $1,000 to officially secure my slot. Of course, one can't expect too much fanfare. The celebration is Kona. It's where I would celebrate all that was achieved through belief, massive action, pain, passion, and perseverance.

I had qualified. I had done it legitimately. I had gone from the very bottom of depravity, fear, and hopelessness to become one of the top amateur triathletes in the world. It was a massive transformation created by breaking myself down into the smallest, most vulnerable parts and piecing myself back together again while learning to become the person I wanted to be. Qualifying for Kona didn't make me who I was. It was the trial and error, the pain, the joy, and everything else that led up to it.

After Mike Riley announced the first two names in my age group to qualify, he called my name. I don't remember him saying my name. I do remember leaping up to accept before he could even get the words out, but the rest is kind of a blur. A cheap, yet priceless, plastic flower lei was placed around my neck, and I was given a coin to commemorate the achievement. The coin had a picture of the Big Island on it. Fitting, since the action taken to get to this point could only be described as "big."

In less than three months, I would be racing mere meters from where I had relapsed back into the depths of alcoholism. Racing in places where I had, at one time, drank heavily, felt poetic and healing. It gave me a new appreciation for those places as the beauty of my present life began to outshine the pain of my past. First, it was Cabo San Lucas, where I drank my way through the bars and into blackouts. Then it was Sonoma, where I would come to drink wine more heavily than one should while wine tasting. In both these places, I later crossed the iconic finish line of an extreme endurance sport, and I did so as a sober person at the peak of fitness and health.

Kona would be one more opportunity to make amends with a place that was once dark to me. It was one more chance to heal and transcend the wreckage of my past and fortify the person I had become. I wasn't going to win the race in Kona. I wasn't even going to make the podium. I would probably finish somewhere in the middle of the pack. Hell, I could even finish dead last. Regardless of where I finished on that day, or how hard it would be, it was going to be a victory.

DID I TELL YOU I
RACED KONA?

THE IRONMAN WORLD CHAMPIONSHIP, 2017.
KAILUA-KONA, HAWAII. MILE 0.

I was struggling badly with my swim cap and goggles. For some reason, I just couldn't get them over my freshly shaved head as I stood elbow-to-elbow with the world's best athletes, all corralling slowly into the calm waters of Kailua Bay. I was doing my best not to look scared shitless as a camera focused intently on my face. I knew that the cameraman was trying to get that one hint of anxiety, a single bead of sweat, a small tremor, or hyperventilation to signify my terror as I prepared to swim the 2.4 miles into the ocean of Hawaii to begin the race I dreamed about doing for the last four years.

I tried hard to don my best poker face for the nationwide audience, but I failed miserably at looking brave. Three failed attempts to put on my swim cap only amplified that point. One attempt sent my cap into a German man, who looked mildly irritated. He would probably not hesitate to punch me hard in the face in a few minutes.

In the days leading up to the race, my anxiety reached all-time highs. Seeing this race on TV and experiencing it are two entirely different things. The insane amount of energy around the island, the "bigness" of everything (including the swells), and all the training that I had been doing for the last few years led to conflicting sensations.

This is freaking awesome! I thought. *Don't fuck it up!*

I had pushed through the anxiety in the days leading up to the race and devised a plan to overcome the fear on race day, a practice that had successfully seen me through many anxiety attacks in the past. As the Boy Scouts always say, "Be prepared."

I ended up writing down some of the worst-case scenarios associated with a race swim, along with all of the safety measures, contingency plans, and likely scenarios that would happen. Worst case scenario: I start to drown. Reality: Nobody has ever died in the Ironman World Championship swim. There are paddleboarders and kayakers every fifty to one hundred meters. Saltwater is super buoyant. I have completed the distance many times, and I am a much fitter swimmer than many of the athletes competing.

This exercise really helps me overcome any specific anxiety attack I may have at any given moment. Most of the time, we are overreacting, and the likely case is far more tolerable than the worst case.

It was with these gentle reminders that I left the safety of the small patch of sand on Dig Me Beach and ventured off toward the uncertainty of the in-water mass swim start. The hundred-meter swim to the start line was calm and easy, and the fear was lifted.

As I found my place behind the pack of confident swimmers who would be punching and kicking their way through the next hour, I was overcome by a merciful calm. This is what I had been striving to achieve for the last four years. I went from a person who had no business doing an Ironman to an elite athlete racing in the world championship. It was an ending to that journey, yet it was also a beginning to new adventures to come. It would be a point of reference for things I had yet to achieve but never believed that I could. The cannon, which was about to fire, would start a victory lap of epic proportions, and when I would cross the finish line somewhere between nine and seventeen hours later, it would be a new beginning.

In the year to come, long after the suffering, physical pain, and euphoria of this race faded into my memory, I would find equilibrium in my life again. I would find balance with work and life, build a coaching platform, and continue to develop my talents as an athlete. Yet my mind wasn't on any of that at this moment. I was simply taking in the whole experience, living in the present moment, looking around me at all of the iconic scenes, and willing them into my memory.

I thought back on the moment that my life changed forever. My bottom. The point that could have been a tragedy of my own making but instead became the catalyst for positive transformation. I thought to myself, *Should I feel ashamed of who I was or grateful that a bad situation led me to become who I am?*

I've learned through experience with sobriety and anxiety that shame is not a productive emotion. It's an emotion people may wish on others who caused destruction, but shame only brings more ruin and hopelessness. Instead of shame, we should seek a genuine willingness to change and transcend our previous destructive patterns. We should take daily massive action in the direction of the person we want to become. We should seek to forgive ourselves and make amends for the harm we have caused. Only then can we begin to heal and grow.

The sun began to peek over Mauna Loa and cast a blinding reflection on the waves breaking over the Kona coast, an indication that the day we were about to face would be hot and windy. Now I was in the water. Now I was committed. There was no turning back, but I looked around with gratitude at the magic that surrounded me. All the visions that were iconic to me from the NBC broadcast of this race—the inflatable Gatorade bottle, the helicopters overhead, the throngs of people littering the seawall and pier, the clear and calm blue waters before me, the thousands of elite triathletes around me, were no longer just fragments of a pipedream. They were a part of a reality that I had manifested through unwavering belief and hard work. My confidence surged with the morning swell. All the racers crept forward as we waited for the cannon.

Whatever was next, I was ready for it. In this race and beyond...

BOOM!

AUTHOR'S NOTE

There are many programs available to help people get sober, and it's not my intention to advocate any single one. For the purposes of illustrating my experience, I chose to divulge that I immersed myself in the twelve-step program of AA since it was such a pivotal part of my story and transformation. This was important to me for a number of reasons. First, I tried the program before, and saw it work for people. I met successfully sober people who found a peace I previously thought was not achievable. Second, my previous attempts were half-assed, at best. My failure was mostly due to not surrendering to an effective recovery program. This time, I did not want to give up without giving it everything I had.

Most importantly, I needed support. I needed mentorship. Working through the steps with someone else helped guide me through the process of my spiritual awakening. It cleared away the fog of my shitty perspective and opened my eyes to a brand-new life. A life full of hope.

The change in perspective was key for me early in sobriety. I learned we all have the ability to shape our own perspectives. Perspective shapes our attitude and outlook, and what's more, it's completely in our control. The people I latched on to in recovery held strong positive outlooks. In every situation, they pointed their perspective toward the positive. When asked how their days were going, they would respond by saying, "I've never had it so good!" They would continuously talk about the grace—or unmerited favor—that they experienced. I was thoroughly intrigued by this attitude, and it was something I desperately wanted.

If I could be transformed in the same way that these optimistic alcoholics could be, maybe I had a chance. I learned early on to find people who had something that I wanted and then do what they told me. Sure enough, that's what I did.

Alcoholics Anonymous is famous for being, well, anonymous. For that reason, I did not go into specific detail about my experiences in AA, lest I compromise some of their core traditions. On the other hand, many of these experiences were critical to my early sobriety, and it's important that I share them as they relate to my experience. Just understand that I did so with respect to the anonymity and traditions of the program of AA. Thus, names, professions, and insignificant details have been changed or omitted.

ACKNOWLEDGMENTS

It is impossible to undertake a significant transformation, let alone write a book about it, without the love, support, encouragement, and inspiration of a tribe of beautiful souls. The most beautiful soul I know is my wife, Marie. Patient, loving, honest, and encouraging; you gave me the spirit and confidence to pursue my dreams and actually believe that I could accomplish them. For the many times you have told me to "Go for it," I thank you. Your grace is the spark that empowered me to become the person I am today.

My children, Sarah and Zachary, have changed my world and given new meaning to my life. They also inspire and amaze me every day. Thank you both for being my support crew at so many races, being an unwilling audience for my dad jokes, and continuing to show me the meaning of joy as you develop into amazing humans.

I recognize how privileged I am to have two parents who love each other deeply and extend that love to their children unconditionally. The seed of passion was planted early in my life, and it was in large part fed by the support and love given to me by Claudia and Ronald Hill. Though I didn't often show enough appreciation early in life, you gave me everything I needed to be successful. I can only hope to pass that grace on to my children as well.

There are many people who have contributed greatly to my growth in sobriety who I cannot name. Yet they are my heroes. They had something I wanted—sobriety—and helped me to discover a solution that ignited a transformation. This is especially true of my sponsor. Thank you for challenging me to look deep inside and change the person I was into the person I wanted to be.

Sharm Luehmann knows me better than I know myself. She is one of very few people who have been with me in darkness and during my best days. At my lowest, she was patient and caring. In my recovery, she guided me on a path of healing. At my best, she helped me discover anxiety as a superpower. Thank you, Sharm, for helping me to see the miracles and possibilities a life of sobriety could bring, and for continuing to be an integral part of my mental health.

I have Calvin Lefebvre to thank for not only helping me recover from my stupid pre-triathlon injuries and the resulting surgeries, but also for giving me the initial guidance I needed to take the first steps on my triathlon journey.

When I first started researching triathlons, I was immediately inspired by Mark Allen and his training philosophy. I was thrilled to take my first steps in this amazing sport under the guidance of his coaching program and partner coach, Luis Vargas. Thank you for making your resources available so that I could learn to level up my fitness and make it to the finish line of my first Ironman Triathlon, and beyond.

I doubt very highly that I would have ever achieved my dream of qualifying for the Ironman World Championship if Eban Hathaway hadn't taken a chance on me. Thank you, Eban, for seeing something worth documenting in me, for cutting out all the embarrassing parts, and for becoming a part of our family. What I am most grateful for in your selection of me for the documentary series is our friendship that came out of it.

Speaking of friends that came out of *Ironman: Quest for Kona*, my fellow castmates became my tribe throughout the process of the documentary series. We encouraged each other, celebrated each other, and became family. To my friends Grace Stevens, Roberto Vieira, Andrew Jamieson, Heather Jenson, A. J. Lane, Eric Beach, Susanne Vanzijl, Rupert Chen, and Maria Teresa "Flaca" Guerrero, you have my gratitude.

Oh...and Susanne, thank you for calming my ass down on the pier before the race in Kona. It was a thrill gawking at super-human triathletes on the Kona pier with you before we joined them for a little race around the Big Island.

A special thank you goes to my very good friend and castmate Eric Beach. In the time since *QFK*, you have always been there for me, to hear out my crazy ideas, read early iterations of this book, advise me on life, and give me honest feedback about all of it. You are not just a friend to me but a hero and a champion.

One of the most important turning points in my life was when I met my best friend, Bryn DuBois. Bryn was there for the formative years of my life and helped to shape my character, my humor, and my confidence. Bryn, thank you for saving my life and for being my confidant, my partner in humor, and my bandmate.

I would not have been able to produce this book without the help of the team at Scribe Media. Thank you to Neddie Ann Underwood for keeping me on task, organized, and steering me in the right direction away from ideas that might have been too crazy. Thank you also to Derek George for designing a great cover, and to Nicole Jobe and Mckenna Bailey for helping me clarify my voice.

I also want to thank those that helped me early in the book publishing process. To Andi Cumbo-Floyd, thank you for your feedback on my earliest draft and for your recommendations on how I could improve the story. That feedback made a huge difference. To Sarah Fox of The Bookish Fox, thank you for the thorough copyedit and storyline suggestions. You helped sharpen my story so that it was ready for prime time.

Finally, thank you to the triathlon community for welcoming me into your tribe. It truly is a remarkable community, and I'm grateful that we all have the opportunity to lift up and inspire one another.